Contents

Occupational Health

FOR MARJORY

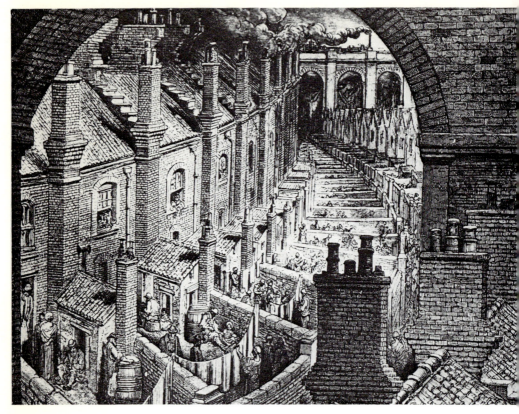

Frontispiece Victorian "back-to-backs", and still with us. (*from "London Pilgrimage" by Gustav Doré, London 1872*).

Occupational Health

Dr. Geoffrey Ffrench

MTP
Medical and Technical Publishing Co. Ltd.

Published by
MTP
Medical and Technical Publishing Co Ltd
St Leonard's House, St Leonardgate
Lancaster, England

SBN 852 000 64 2

Printed in Great Britain by
Billing & Sons Limited, Guildford and London

30/1/90

Foreword

"HOLD THOU THE GOOD: DEFINE IT WELL . . ."

The quotation above from Tennyson, is apt when describing the purpose and achievement of this book.

The author is dedicated to his subject – personal health in industry: his research covers practical experience in the U.K. and other lands.

In non-technical language the book records many of the causes of ill-health and throws light upon the physical and mental stress with which men and women at work have to contend.

Dr. Ffrench's observations and conclusions should be of considerable value to employers of labour and of interest to all concerned in the welfare of people engaged in earning a living.

HAROLD COOPER
Alfred H. Cooper & Sons Ltd

Preface

This book has been prepared so that readers may appreciate the significant change in attitudes which has taken place over the past twenty-five years towards the care of the health of people at work. Ideally it should be read in conjunction with such handbooks as those by Harvey and Murray, and Browne which emphasise the care that should be given toward the physical aspects of the work environment. I have not attempted to cover the ground again. Of equal importance are the psychological stresses which people meet at their work and the interplay these have with the more traditional aspects of the occupational environment. Therefore I have attempted a personal appraisal of those situations met every day by millions of people in this country. In doing so I am fully aware that not all the views and opinions expressed will meet with full acceptance by readers, whether these are my colleagues or those in government or industry whose responsibility it is to provide occupational health services. Nevertheless, I hope that what I have said will stimulate some discussion but, more purposefully, positive action to widen the field of preventive measures to protect the total health of people at work. That this attitude is not restricted to those with what has euphemistically been called "missionary zeal", I quote from a recent statement made by the Division of Occupational Health of the Government of New South Wales in Australia: "We have now reached the stage when it is felt to be insufficient simply to save the worker from severe disability or death. We must concern ourselves with his 'health' in the widest sense of the word. As the World Health Organisation puts it, our objective should be to promote his 'physical mental, and social well-being'. It is with the more subtle stresses, those which produce discomfort rather than serious injury, that ergonomics is mainly concerned."

GEOFFREY FFRENCH

Acknowledgements

I am grateful for the help I have received from a host of people who must remain anonymous. They comprise my patients and colleagues, medical and non-medical, with whom I have shared experience over the years in the air, on the ground and under the ground. They have shown me the pleasures and pitfalls of man management as well as allowing me their confidence.

Some portions of this book have appeared elsewhere and I acknowledge my debt to the Editors of *The Lancet*, the *Transactions* (now the *Journal*) *of the Society of Occupational Medicine*, *Industrial Safety*, *District Nursing* and *The Ambulance Bulletin*.

Mr. Harold Cooper, who has been kind enough to contribute a Foreword, has been of great help to me during the five years we have been associated in the Central Middlesex Industrial Health Service, of which he is Chairman.

I would be churlish indeed if I failed to say how much assistance I have received from my wife during the three years this book has taken us.

1 Introduction

Ancient Man, the hunter and gatherer of nuts and herbs, was himself the natural prey of his carnivorous animal neighbours; no doubt he had considerable reluctance in accepting this state of affairs. In time, however, he discovered that by the better co-ordinated use of his forelimbs he could fashion first weapons and later tools which allowed him to master his enemies and his immediate environment. Thus he learnt to manufacture, to "make with his hands": since then he has never faltered, because of the unique phenomenon of "feed-back" which enabled the brain to develop in response to the message from the hands, in turn guiding the hands to ever greater skills by virtue of the reasoning power developed by the enlarging forebrain.

   The circumstances which have governed the rate and manner of human development have been remarkably varied, for even today there are humans living much as our ancestors did twenty thousand years ago. Probably the one factor above all others which influences human progress is the rate at which people have to adapt and alter their style of living as a result of changes in the natural environment. In historical times there has been an accelerating manipulation of the environment and its products: the pace of these changes resulting from natural phenomena can be measured over thousands of years. When man first began to use his hands the innovations resulting were timed on this scale: but once he was past the Iron Age, which took him about 500,000 years to reach, there was no stopping him. We must accept that the first anatomical type of pre-man appeared about half a million years ago in the deep forest areas of Africa and South-east Asia. He did not develop into the Homo sapiens we ourselves are today until about 20,000 years ago, and then it was along two world planes, one North African or Mediterranean, the other

North European and Siberian. If we plot the change over these 20,000 years we can judge the rate of advance which, in the last fifty years is threatening, by its acceleration, to overwhelm man's natural ability to adapt and acclimatise himself to the changes, for time is of the essence in order to do this. There do not appear as yet to be any means of controlling the superabundance of technology; these are desperately needed.

Any student of the ancient craft of tool-making must become aware of the enormity of the hazards to which ancient man was exposed in his daily work, whether these were fire, fumes or festering wounds. There is a surprising amount of discerning observation in Greek literature of the damaging effects of mechanical labour upon the human body, referring particularly to the hapless labourers in mine and foundry: to these we can add the effects upon the lungs of the dusts raised from quarrying and pottery. Hippocrates (fifth century B.C.), the "Father of Medicine", observed, with masterly insight, the appalling conditions in which people worked; he impressed upon his students the need to consider all the environmental factors when making a diagnosis on a patient. He made particular reference to the poisoning of refiners and extractors of metals. The Romans later gave us an expression we still sometimes use when describing a gloomy man – we say he has a "saturnine look" about him, which describes the dull pallor of his skin and the depressed and morose appearance of his countenance. Saturnism was the term applied by Roman physicians to the effects of lead poisoning, for lead was known by the word saturn for many hundreds of years due to its ability to alloy with other metals, or as the ancients thought, to "consume and absorb them". Another colloquialism, "mad as a hatter", was at one time thought to refer to a well-known form of poisoning, this time mercury, and stems from the not uncommon mental effects of mercury poisoning characteristic of the felt hat-making industry in England and elsewhere during the nineteenth century. It has been said, though without foundation, that the character of the Hatter in Lewis Carroll's *Alice's Adventures in Wonderland* was modelled on the quarrelsome, sensitive yet timid individual with poor self-control, the so-called erethism characteristic of chronic mercury posioning: the term more rightly derives from the older expression "mad as an adder" (*Talking Sense* by Richard Asher, Pitman, London, 1972, p. 179). The Felt-hat Manufacture Regulations (1902), still serve to remind us of this formerly not uncommon illness. Despite these and many similar observations relating cause and effect in working environments, little was done, until the nineteenth century, to mitigate them. The very cheapness and availability of labour, together with a stoic accept-

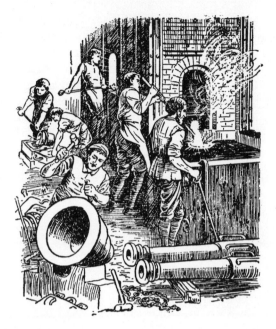

Fig. 1 A 17th-century cannon forge in the Kentish Weald (*from "Wealden Exploration" by Roger A. B. Castle, Tunbridge Wells, 1971*).

ance of illness and death, combined to retard measures to identify the causes of illness and combat their effects. No better descriptions have been given than by Agricola (George Bauer) (1494–1555) who recorded both the nature and methods of the mining and refining industries together with their effects upon the luckless workers during the sixteenth century in the industrial areas of southern Germany and Bohemia. These activities antedated the English Industrial Revolution by over two hundred years. It is worth recalling that in Europe, including Britain, during the centuries preceding the discovery of coal and steam, industry was distributed over the countryside in close proximity to great woods and forests, the only practical source of fuel. These centres became the origin of many of the great towns of the Middle Ages not all of which have survived: others continued to prosper long after their forests had disappeared. No better example of this can be given than the industrial activities centred upon the Weald of Kent and Sussex, and again in the West Country. The remains of this pre-coal industry are found often only in name, the physical presence having disappeared under some of the most productive and beautiful agricultural land in the world. Today, throughout the country new products are constantly being introduced and used in homes, in gardens and on the

land: new hazards are arising, old ones remain. The pattern of
modern urban development is now once again the establishment of
light industry adjacent to towns and villages: thus the concept of
occupational health is broadening to include many occupations
outside of the factory, in hospitals, universities, colleges and laboratories, impinging on many who had not previously considered its
significance in their own lives. To this end the following chapters are
devoted.

2 Health at Work

THE WORKING ENVIRONMENT

Successful adaptation to environment has so far been the hallmark of the human animal. This adaptation begins *in utero*, although the foetus is protected from minor physical insults by the insulating medium of the amniotic fluid. As soon as this has been discarded, hard surfaces and sometimes hard people commence the process in earnest and the rest of life is taken up with developing defences and reactions to an enormous variety of physical and psychological influences, exemplified, among others, by immunological and neurotic responses, evidence of which we all possess. Whilst heredity and environment probably play an equal part in intellectual and physical development, environmental challenges are absolutely necessary for the development of maturity.

Taking the whole span of a person's life, the working environment is the most consistent and impressive of these challenges, or at least it has the potential of being so. Nevertheless, because of the additive effects of the whole life experience, particularly family and formal education, no one of these can be considered in isolation. This should be the keynote of our attitude towards occupational health, for people every day are experiencing a far greater variety of working environments than the more restricted pattern of their domestic life allows. One half of the time a person is not engaged in sleeping is taken up by gainful employment stretching frequently over forty or more years. With the reintroduction of women into industry following the 1914–18 War and the subsequent expansion of light assembly, textile and packaging, to name but a few outlets, women have become a major factor in the work-force of this country, comprising slightly more than half the total full and part-time labour force of

26 million. I said "reintroduction of women" because it should be recalled that large numbers of women worked in indescribable conditions prior to the enactment of factory legislation in the nineteenth century. But women's work does not cease on re-entering the home, and this may have some bearing in the greater sickness absence frequency in women workers. Patterns of work are changing for both men and women: for some, hours are shortening, and second jobs are increasing; for others overtime is becoming a regular theme; and yet others are engaging in hobbies, handicrafts and exhausting sporting activities which may have their dangers. All of these must be taken into account when assessing the whole life situation.

Satisfaction at work has been a traditional experience. When manual labour predominated, each and every one "knew their station in life" and received recognition of their work. Today this is no longer true and many thousands of people are not experiencing a sense of challenge and appreciation for their work. The more demanding and challenging work is, the greater the satisfaction; the less the obstacles to surmount by the introduction of mechanisation, the more the sense of personal obsolescence and insignificance, leading to boredom and frustration. The factors which govern satisfaction with a job depend very much on the education an individual has gained in his pre-work experience and the training he received for the job he is to do; the design of the work and the way it is to be done must fit the capacity of both healthy and disabled people. A balance must be struck between the desire for work and the optimum social security.

SCOPE OF OCCUPATIONAL HEALTH

Some of the many factors that influence the prevalence of symptoms and the sickness patterns of individuals and families are undoubtedly related to the working environment; to take an extreme though real example is the recognition of the care required that asbestos workers should free themselves and their clothes of any residual asbestos before returning home. Exposure to asbestos by family members has resulted in the development of malignant mesothelioma, a cancer of the covering membrane of the lung.

Occupational health can be said to be the creation of a state of physical and mental well-being, within the occupational environment, while taking into consideration factors relating to the social and domestic life of each individual. This broad definition exceeds the limited responsiblities of the Factories Acts and comes well within the field of the general practitioner's responsibility for the total health of his population. This implies a broader responsibility than that of the doctor working in isolation: if he can see himself as a member of a team covering all the sectors of health, preventive, curative, educational and welfare, then with co-ordinated effort, occupational health should fall naturally into place. In urban and suburban areas, many people live and have their social life at some distance from their working environment and it is difficult for the family doctor to become aware of the occupational conditions of his patients. Similarly, those responsible for health care within industry do not know the social and domestic background of their workers. Nevertheless, the family doctor, by possessing a general knowledge of working environments and their significance to health, together with a channel to more specialised information, can make the tasks of early recognition of disorder and prevention easier, not only in his own patient, but also in the working conditions of others.

THE POSITION IN BRITAIN

Compared to the outstanding developments in other fields of public health and general medicine, occupational health has been relatively neglected in Britain. The International Labour Organisation in Geneva, the active offspring of the now defunct League of Nations, has, for many years, laid down the principles and requirements for maintaining health at work. Many countries have adopted part or all of these. Furthermore the Treaty of Rome 1957 aims "to promote close collaboration between member states in the social field, particularly in matters relating to . . . protection against occupational accidents and disease . . . industrial hygiene". It also has declared certain principles to be accepted by member countries:

1. That factories employing more than 200 people should provide an occupational health service, preferably by doctors engaged full time in the field of occupational medicine who have received the necessary training.
2. No one doctor should care for more than 2,500 employees.
3. An interim period of six years following membership during which doctors entering or already engaged in occupational health will be required to obtain statutory qualifications.
4. The High Commission of the European Economic Community to be informed, at two-yearly intervals, of the implementation of these recommendations.

Despite Britain's lead in industrial legislation during the nineteenth and early twentieth centuries, we have not yet accepted these principles. It remains to be seen whether we will do so in 1973.
Since the first Act of Parliament designed to protect the "health

NOTICE

TO EMPLOYEES

1. Godliness, cleanliness and punctuality are the necessities of a good business.
2. This firm has reduced the hours of work, and the clerical staff will now only have to be present between the hours of 7 a.m. and 6 p.m. on weekdays.
3. Daily prayers will be held each morning in the main office. The clerical staff will be present.
4. Clothing must be of a sober nature. The clerical staff will not disport themselves in raiment of bright colours, nor will they wear hose, unless in good repair.
5. Overshoes and top-coats may not be worn in the office, but neck scarves and headwear may be worn in inclement weather.
6. A stove is provided for the benefit of the clerical staff. Coal and wood must be kept in the locker. It is recommended that each member of the clerical staff bring in 4 pounds of coal each day during cold weather.
7. No member of the clerical staff may leave the room without permission from Mr. Rogers. The calls of nature are permitted and the clerical staff may use the garden below the second gate. This area must be kept in good order.
8. No talking is allowed during business hours.
9. The craving for tobacco, wines or spirits is a human weakness and as such is forbidden to all members of the clerical staff.
10. Now that the hours of business have been so drastically reduced, the partaking of food is only allowed between 11.30 a.m. and noon, but work will not, on any account, cease.
11. Members of the clerical staff will provide their own pens. A new sharpener is available, on application to Mr. Rogers.
12. Mr. Rogers will nominate a senior clerk to be responsible for the cleanliness of the main office and the private office, and all boys and juniors will report to him 40 minutes before prayers, and will remain after closing hours for similar work. Brushes, brooms, scrubbers and soap are provided by the owners.
13. The new increased weekly wages are as hereunder detailed: Junior boys (up to eleven years) 1s. 4d., Boys (to 14 years) 2s. 1d., Juniors 4s. 8d., Junior clerks 8s. 7d., Clerks 10s. 9d., Senior Clerks (after 15 years with owners) 21s.

The owners recognise the generosity of the new Labour Laws, but will expect a great rise in output of work to compensate for these near utopian conditions.

Office regulations for a Burnley cotton mill in 1852.

Fig. 2 (*Courtesy of Bri-Mer Company, London.*)

and morals of apprentices" in 1802 there has been a steady series of Factories Acts related to special fields of health and hygiene in industry, but it was not until the Act of 1896 that the appointment of the first medical inspector of factories was made. In 1891 medical examinations of young people had been introduced, although fifty years earlier, in 1844, the first certifying factory surgeon had been appointed to ensure that children and young persons were not made unfit by their work. Only in 1901 were these doctors permitted to examine the place of work, enabling them to qualify and support their opinions.

At no time has any employer in this country, except certain government industries in wartime and since, been required to provide an occupational medical service of a more comprehensive nature than is needed under the various Acts: even these are limited to specific environmental hazards and minimum hygiene standards. Many of the obscure and insidious environmental problems of industrial and indeed all forms of work fall outside the statutory requirements and are often left unsought and uncared for. This is the position today for some 90 per cent of the 26 million full-and part-time British workers. This situation shows no sign of being abated by government action; efforts by some industrialists since the end of the eighteenth century have reduced work load, improved health and provided a medical advisory service at their factories. Today there are some medical services in British industry second to none, but these apply to no more than a small percentage of the working population. Another 7 or 8 per cent receive some form of medical and health care of variable quality, ranging from those factories and organisations which are members of a group industrial health service to part-time attendance by nursing officers or doctors who are not required by law to have any special training for the work. The situation is not easy for employers. If the factory employs many people, it may financially justify the retention of full- or part-time medical staff, whose terms of reference can vary widely depending upon the views of the employers and, we would like to think, of the employees and relevant trade unions. Both the latter have, up till now, taken remarkably little part in the demand for or provision of these services. But the smaller firms, who may employ from 10 to 250 workers, have a problem in justifying the expense of such a service.

WHAT IS NEEDED?

Until the publication of the Robens Committee's report on the health and safety of people at work in 1972, there had been no clear indication of the future patterns and no government department has been willing to take responsibility for developing an integrated occupational or industrial medical service. While the trade unions are very concerned, it has been left to the initiative of the larger industries which make up less than 10 per cent of the working force to set up their own services and for certain local areas to follow on a smaller scale.

The structure of an occupational health service will vary with the needs of the industry and working group concerned, depending upon known and potential industrial environmental problems, the predominance of certain age and sex groups and geographical considerations such as isolation from emergency services.

After World War II a start was made on the needs of the host of small industries employing under 250 people by providing co-operative group industrial health services to furnish advice and emergency treatment which could not otherwise be obtained on an acceptable economic basis. These services, situated at Slough, Harlow, North-west London (Central Middlesex), West Birmingham, Rochdale, Dundee and Newcastle, at present cater for some 100,000 workers, a tiny fraction of the country's total work-force. The opportunity to create further services is greatly reduced now that the very generous support of the Nuffield Foundation, without which the first six could have not made a start, is no longer available. At today's costs, about £50,000 is required to capitalise a unit and a work-force of at least 5,000 must be recruited for financial viability.

Group general practices and health centres have encouraged the sharing of responsibilities and enabled doctors to develop wider interests and the opportunity to improve the overall quantity and quality of medical services to the local community. Occupational health should be included among those wider interests. The new health centres could provide both the nursing and auxiliary staff so essential to occupational health, together with the emergency facilities now being given by the group industrial health services.

For this pattern of service to be provided, there must be a general acknowledgement that a medical advisory service should be available to the worker during the working day to achieve a "quick turn-round", to borrow an industrial phrase. The recent trend for the abolition of late evening surgeries, in itself an excellent thing for family doctors and clinic staff, has tacitly acknowledged this need by failing to provide alternative hours outside the working period: this has led to the use of other available services, casualty departments of hospitals and industrial medical services. Some system of integrating them with general medical practice on the lines discussed should be seriously examined in every industrial area by the existing community health authorities.

To summarise we can say that a knowledge of the working environment is paramount in interpreting the health needs of people at work. The possibility of this environment being a causal factor should be considered at the general practitioner's first contact with an adult patient.

The scope of occupational health extends not only to the requirements of the Factories Act, but far beyond into an understanding of the functional and psychological requirements of people while at work and in their domestic and social milieu.

A brief mention has been made of international requirements, our own national legislation and the limited steps taken independently beyond these minimum requirements by employers. Suggestions have been made as to how responsibility for occupational health can be shared by doctors and paramedical workers within the community.

3 People at Work

CONDITIONS AT WORK

As the quality and design of plant and buildings improve so should the working environment, but if anybody doubts that unacceptable conditions of dirt and dust, sweat, stink and noise continue to exist, let him visit the narrow, dark alleys and railway arches where small enterprises produce a wide variety of metal and plastic products many of which are components of machines and consumer goods with household names. It is under these conditions that bizarre and traditional forms of industrial accidents and intoxications still arise: while one might hope that such conditions may become things of the past, this is unlikely. The Factories Inspectorate is not in a position to cover all the potential risks frequently enough to ensure safety.

The growing numbers of women in industry and the full recognition of their value when weighed against the statutory requirements of the Factories Act have highlighted the importance of the working space, the light and the air they breathe. The last reported figures, in 1964, of men and women workers in England and Wales *who were subject to the Factories Act*, were 14·3 and 8 million respectively. The continued improvement in the design of machinery and furniture has contributed to the ability to absorb a wider group of people, to include the older worker, the disabled and the problem people inevitable in any collection of individuals, social or industrial.

HEALTH RECORDS

The compilation of occupational health records from a variety of sources is time-consuming and expensive; their maintenance and constant up-dating a further charge. The justification for this expense can be made only in the long term. One may take the examples of some at-risk groups such as those agricultural workers using potentially dangerous organo-phosphorus insecticides, the sewer workers in an urban community, the carding-room workers in a cotton-mill and abattoir workers. These are a few of the people who may constitute a significant proportion of a local community either in numbers or by the potential effects of their work. In this respect then it would be helpful if general practitioners had some personal knowledge of the local industries.

THE DISTRIBUTION OF WORKERS

There is now general agreement among demographers that Britain is over-populated, but there are still not enough workers of the required skill; either they live in the wrong places and will not migrate, or, for a number of reasons not necessarily related to industrial organisation, they are restless and do not remain long in their job. This generates a high turnover together with the difficulty and expense of training, with resulting loss of production. To remedy this situation foreign immigrant workers have to be brought in, a solution not unique to Britain. Some of our commercial rivals, notably France, Sweden and Germany, share these frustrations; but this is not a novel phenomenon, although the extent of the demand and the social effects are a new experience.

Successive waves of refugees and true migrants originally stimulated the development of certain industries in this country, which in turn led to further demand for skilled workers. Well-known examples are the development of silk, glass and paper manufacturing following the settlement of many thousands of Huguenots from France after the revocation of the Edict of Nantes in 1685, which made the life of the French Protestants unbearable. By one stroke of the pen Louis XIV removed the core of the manufacturing potential of France and gave England her chance to develop almost unchallenged, for at that time the rest of Europe was still on its knees with exhaustion after the Thirty Years War (1619–48). It is significant that coincidentally in England there developed a great leap forward in scientific and industrial experiment, invention and expansion which antedated what we usually consider the Industrial Revolution by more than a hundred years. For instance, it was at this time that the first practical steam engine was developed by Newcomen which in turn led to the further expansion of coal-mining by providing the motive power to pump water out of the mines; it also created the sudden demand for a cheap labour force. This example of the industrial

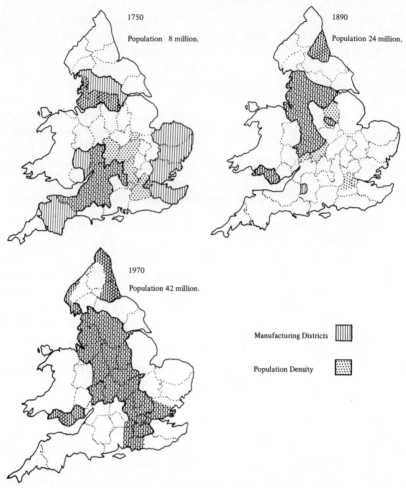

Fig. 3 Manufacturing districts and population density in England over the past 200 years. Initially there was a shift of population to the North and North-west but this has now returned to the Midlands and South-east.

"pull" stimulating immigration was echoed in the Irish migrations of the nineteenth century, and the steady procession from Britain's former colonies and dominions over the past twenty years. The relative impact on this country has been comparable. At the time of the Huguenot immigration England's population was 8,000,000: at mid-point of the nineteenth century 16,000,000 and in 1970 42,000,000. Place the immigration figures against these population totals and the proportions are much the same, although the effect now is more striking due to overall increase of population density in certain geographical areas. At each of these periods of immigration Britain has profited to the extent that its production potential and technology has been considerably augmented during periods of high demand. In less prosperous times the case is altered.

But the problems of regional and international migration bear heavily upon the work of community health, industrial management, personnel relations and the welfare services of local government. While some areas of the country remain free of migration, others are almost transformed, relating in the main to the demand for labour.

The mixture of races that comprise the British people has given them a toughness and resilience tested time and again over the past thousand years. The infusion of exotic genes has had an overall beneficial effect, whether the source was swarthy Syrian legionaries of the Roman army of occupation, red-headed Norsemen intent upon pillage or stolid Flemings from the Low Countries who came to put our wool textile industry on its feet in the seventeenth century. True, there have been occasional genetic "accidents" which can be traced back to foreign elements of which perhaps the best examples with us today are familial periodic paralysis of Scandinavian origin, and the rare haemoglobinopathies (disorders of oxygen-carrying haemoglobin in the red blood cells) probably from the Mediterranean basin and the Middle East. In the future we can expect to see more of these, particularly the haemoglobinopathies and the enzyme disorders affecting the red blood cells, for many of the people now entering our population are carriers of these traits, originally developed as protective mechanisms against malaria. With the exposure of such people to the processes and emissions of modern industry there is a possibility that their health could suffer disproportionately. This is a field only just beginning to be explored but illustrates the importance of knowing something of the human material and its fallibility.

INFORMATION SERVICES

Coupled with the local knowledge of demand for labour, familiarity with the different local industries and their distribution among heavy and light engineering, assembly, food, plastics, packaging, etc. is useful, and here the co-operation of government departments in supplying information of this nature should be sought by planners, employers and those responsible for occupational health services. At the present time no such information is routinely made available, among others, to general practitioners who could benefit greatly. The only source is the Factories Inspectorate and they are not authorised to provide or up-date such information beyond their own needs. This emphasises the need for co-ordinated community information services.

RETIREMENT

Full-time employment on the whole is restricted to between the ages of 16 and 65, while part-time work is not covered by legislation. It is now becoming evident that the curtailing of work beyond 65 has brought with it problems for the individual and for society. The approach to retirement and its reality to anyone not intellectually gifted or possessing adaptability and opportunities for continued though modified productive work can be traumatic. This has been recognised for some years by the introduction of pre-retirement adaptation and retraining for post-retirement occupation. Flexibility in the structure of employment could lead to considerable easing of this problem, particularly for those who have the capability and motivation to continue working. This subject will be discussed in some detail later in this book.

THE CROSS-CULTURAL OUTLOOK

The social structure of a general practice may vary widely, depending upon its location, the population it is designed to serve and, not least, the doctor who runs it. This is particularly relevant in the new-town practices which may have a preponderance of social groups or classes III, IV, V. This social structure has a bearing on the attitudes of the doctor in the community. Most important is that he should appreciate the differences between people and groups of people, their cultures and interests and, not least, his own discrepancies. Maurice King has emphasised this in relation to work in developing

TABLE 1

SOCIAL CLASS	DEFINITION
1	The Professional Occupations
2	Intermediate
3	The Skilled Occupations
4	Intermediate
5	The Unskilled Occupations

Table of Social Classes (or Groups) as used by the Registrar General: "they are necessarily arbitrary and reflect standing in the Community rather than economic levels".

Taylor I., Knowelden J. Principles of Epidemiology. London 1964/336.

countries, whether the doctor be indigenous or expatriate: the value of the "cross-cultural" outlook cannot be over-stressed.

In the traditional picture of general practice in former days the social classes were perhaps more clearly defined; more authority was vested in the doctor by virtue of knowledge possessed solely by himself, and thus his task was made easier to the extent that his patients did not question his judgement and knowledge; neither was there the demanding attitude related to benefits under social and medical welfare legislation. Still, his task was not easy: his knowledge was limited and his therapeutic tools inadequate. The doctor of today is incomparably better prepared to deal with the physical illness, but in the main still somewhat ill-equipped to handle the psychological and social ills of his patients, thogh he may recognise their significance. Of these, the occupational implications justify an understanding by the physician of the industrial behavioural patterns involving his patients, whether they be in the managerial field or on the shop floor. It should be remembered that, even today, the preparation of the young doctor to appreciate and recognise the interplay of the physical, psychological and social components of disease is still inadequate, and ten years of practice are usually needed before this understanding and experience can be effectively applied to daily problems of diagnosis.

SICKNESS ABSENCE AND CERTIFICATION

It is easy to fall into the trap of regarding a working population as statistical data rather than fallible human beings. Annual sickness rates and lost time have reached high figures and these do not include episodes of three days or less. The British figures relate specifically to the certification given by the general practitioner and he is seen to play a key role in the control of this problem under the present legislation. It is the doctor's perception and ability to gauge the capacity of a patient to return to work which is the one control that this country at present possesses, a control upon which our economic growth and living standards depend. Certification is, however, under severe attack by the medical profession and its value charged with doubt for both sickness frequency and length of sickness spells have almost doubled over the last fifteen years among workers under 45 years of age, while remaining fairly constant in those over 45. Industrial experience of non-certificated spells of sickness of three days or less parallels these findings. It would seem that this phenomenon is subject to the whim and the moral and social demands of a proportion of the workers, analogous to the demand upon a general practitioner's services by a small element of his population.

TABLE 2

OPINIONS EXPRESSED ABOUT THE JOB

GROUP	DEFINITELY ENJOY		INDIFFERENT		DISLIKE JOB	
	No.	%	No.	%	No.	%
Frequently sick	26	46	20	36	10	18
Controls	45	80	9	16	2	4
Long sick	26	74	7	20	2	6
Never sick	45	96	1	2	1	2
All men	142	72	37	20	15	8

SICKNESS ABSENCE AND JOB SATISFACTION

"In this direct assessment of job satisfaction, definite enjoyment of the job was very significantly less common (P. 0·003) in the frequently sick than in the control group. The never sick were almost unanimous in saying that they definitely enjoyed their job. At the other extreme of opinion, only the frequently sick had a significant number of men admitting that they disliked their job (P 0·005)."

(*Peter Taylor "Personal factors Associated with sickness absence". BJIM 25. 106–118. 1968.*)

Certification can be helped, however, by assessing a patient's fitness against the knowledge of the work he does, precisely the situation he would meet were he to return to work at a factory where there is an industrial physician – but too few of our factories or other industrial organisations give themselves the benefit of such a service. The general practitioner with a fair understanding of working environments should be at least partially equipped to consider his patient's request for certification. Doctors in other countries are faced with a similar problem, although it has been very difficult to arrange valid comparisons owing to the different criteria for data collection. Nevertheless, the continued rise in frequency of sickness episodes can be identified, and has been computed to show a mean for all age groups of 34 per cent in Great Britain, West Germany, Italy, Czechoslovakia over seventeen years. On the other hand severity, as identified by length of spells of sickness, rose only 19 per cent over the same period. It will be seen that while the five countries all showed a rise in frequency, only one, Czechoslovakia, revealed a drop in the severity. But this aspect of severity must also occasion us some concern, for by failing to be reduced reciprocally with the rise in frequency, it implies a total increase in the morbidity of the industrial population, assuming that the rates have been standardised for age and sex: the ratios of these are known to have

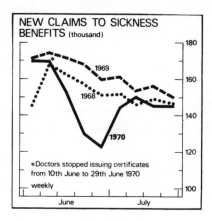

NEW CLAIMS TO SICKNESS
BENEFITS (thousand)

1969

1968

1970

∗Doctors stopped issuing certificates
from 10th June to 29th June 1970

weekly

June   July

Fig. 4 This graph would seem to support the argument that withdrawal of the requirement for doctors to certify short-term sickness would reduce sickness absence wastage. During the 19 days of medical non-cooperation, anyone who claimed sickness benefit had to fill in a special form for his social security office; this made short-term benefit more difficult to obtain. (*Reproduced by permission from "The Economist" September 1970*).

changed over the period in question. That there may be other explanations for this failure of reduction in the length of sickness spells is beyond the border of our present discussion except to say that evidence is accumulating to link both frequency and severity to neurotic and economic as well as medical factors, particularly in the younger ages.

In Sweden and elsewhere suspicions are growing that some of the absenteeism is related to "moonlighting", or the pursuit of a second gainful occupation. The recognition of the disproportionate demand from some patients in a general practice is mirrored by the experience of industry. It is here that the general practitioner can communicate with his patient's work-place to see if his own experience of frequent certification is accompanied by a corresponding number of non-certified absences. If this was the case it would help him to recognise the nature of his patient's problem – medical, social, occupational – or a combination of all three. There is a word for these people, "susceptibles". While the general practitioner is concerned to return the patient to a state of well-being, he may at the same time be in a position to advise the employer of the way this might be accelerated; an easier task if the dialogue can be with an industrial physician or nursing officer.

In review then, the salient points of an approach to the health study of people at work hinge primarily on a knowledge of the working environment, the distribution of different groups of people within industry, including age, sex, race and those requiring special

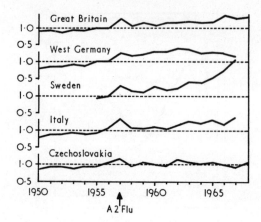

Fig. 5 Sickness frequency ratios. Mean rate 1955 and 1956 = 1·0. (*From "International Trends in Sickness Absence 1950–1968" by P. J. Taylor. Brit. Med. Jour. 4.705-707 1969.*)

care, and adequate recording of attendances, absences and their causes. The relative significance of retirement policies has been touched upon, to be developed later, and the need for a cross-cultural approach to the problem of sickness patterns within a general practice emphasised.

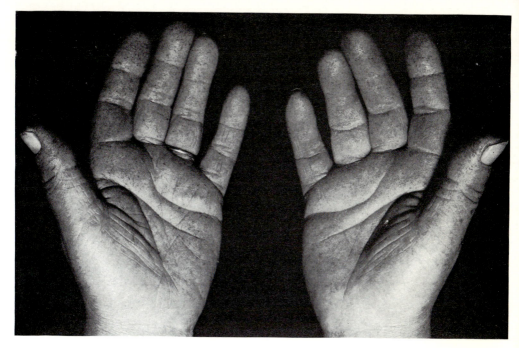

Plate 1 An example of the "hardening" process experienced in some industries: this married woman worked in a close-knit group of four, all of whom had at least twenty years of service in a wire-brush making factory.

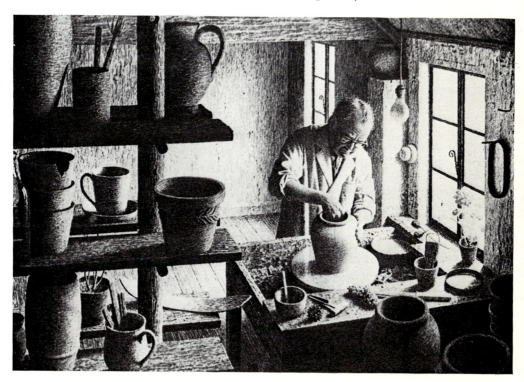

Plate 2 The Craftsman "for in the market-place, one Dusk of Day, I watch'd the potter thumping his wet clay: And with its all obliterated Tongue. It murmur'd – 'Gently, Brother, gently, pray' " (*from the Quatrains of Abolfat'h Ghia'th-E-Din Ebrahim KHAYAM of Nishabur, translated by Edward Fitzgerald*).

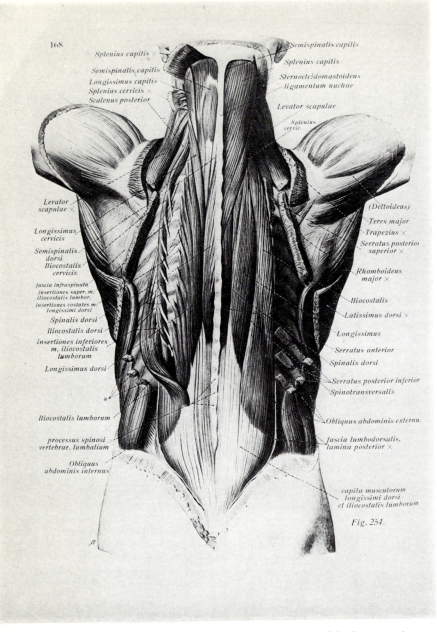

Plate 3 A cut-away representation of the supporting muscles of the human spine and trunk (*from Human Anatomy, Sabotta and McMurrich, New York, 1936, Vol. 1*).

4 The Structure of Management and its Bearing upon Occupational Health

It would be hard to imagine four more diverse characters than: Robert Owen, Lancashire mill-owner and cotton manufacturer, Richard Oastler, Yorkshire land agent, one time inmate of the Fleet prison and reckless orator, Michael Sadler, Tory M.P. for Newark and a rabid anti-Roman Catholic, and Anthony Ashley Cooper, later Lord Shaftesbury, the sensitive and ambitious aristocrat. Yet it was these four men who set the stage for a major social revolution to be enacted during the first fifty years of the nineteenth century; this came about as a result of the appalling conditions arising from the rapid industrialisation of Britain. But it would be less than fair to say that they were the only leaders of a band of industrialists and aristocrats who became aware of the shocking exploitation of men, women and children, and who took the trouble to see with their own eyes what was going on.

It took nearly fifty years of sustained and bitter struggle both in Parliament and throughout the country before many working people were freed from what we would now describe as slavery: these efforts were directly parallelled by those of Wilberforce and his friends engaged in stamping out the more traditional forms of slavery. The story of the struggle and final success is a lesson to us of dogged persistence spiced at times with rabid rebellion, directed to reasonable compromise and the prohibition of human exploitation. These activities must be viewed in the context of the times but they did serve as a template to those industrialists of today who have recognised their social responsibilities towards their employees.

EARLY PIONEERS

Owen's recognition of the influence of the working environment on the health of his employees led him to create what were, at the time, unique industrial communities where the housing and working conditions set an outstanding example to his contemporaries, particularly in the provision of sanitation, schooling and training. But his refusal to employ young children and the payment of unemployment benefit during depressed periods were too far in advance of contemporary practice: these enlightened efforts remained little more than a bold gesture in the face of opposition to his philosophy of communal development and what virtually amounted to the redisposal of profits to improve the welfare of the worker. While his opponents flourished on their short-term success his communities became places of pilgrimage for social reformers and others who were intrigued or curious. The paternalistic nature of this philosophy has had its more contemporary counterparts; Port Sunlight and Bourneville in this country, the Kaiser Corporation in the United States, Badischer Analin Soda Fabrik in Germany and many of the great enterprises which have assisted the awakening of underdeveloped countries. But today the image of paternalism must give way to individual expression and inspiration once the worker has been lifted out of the cradle of good nutrition and education to become willing and able to exert his choice and spend his money himself.

STRESSES ON THE WORKERS

It is salutary that over 150 years after Owen and his fellow campaigners, the task of drawing attention to the need to consider the whole environment of a working man or woman remains a top priority for occupational physicians instead of being reckoned an essential part of standard management practice Why isolate the influence of the working environment when the stresses and pleasures of home and leisure must exert a comparable effect on peace of mind and body and ultimately work performance?

The emphasis now placed on productivity and efficiency has put a burden on the worker which, to the surprise of many, is unrelieved in the majority of instances either by automated assistance or pay increases. The call for greater output means, for some workers, a greater responsibility and greater intensity of application while others experience prolonged boredom to the point of frustration and breakdown which may generate a desire to work discontinuously; this expresses itself by strikes and sickness absenteeism which may provide a cooling-off period and be construed as a therapeutic necessity.

MANAGEMENT AND SPECIALISATION

Management experience has followed closely the paths of other professions, where specialisation has obscured the communications vital to their needs. It is this isolation both in spirit and physical contact which is a strong factor in the distrust between the major working groups, top and middle management and the shop floor. In the past the restriction of engineers and scientists employed in industry to specific technical tasks has assisted this gap to widen. The question now to be answered is whether industry is equipped to handle the challenge to reform: there are many factors to be taken into account. For this reason a review of the structure of management will be helpful.

The definition of manager is of necessity vague, but can be applied to anyone who has responsibility for the work or social activity of others. A "line of management" begins at the top or bottom according to choice and connects "in a line" the managing director and the shop floor, with branches to related advisory technical activities. It requires the twin essentials of administrative and technical ability in balanced proportions. Administration, from an art, has become a technique in itself, involving the understanding of people and personality, industrial psychology, work performance and flow, job analysis, and many other considerations. Industry has made progress in providing facilities for people to study these techniques and the Trades Unions have taken a close interest; but the distribution of this knowledge is uneven, with large numbers of people from the bigger organisations having attended courses and seminars but proportionately less from the smaller firms: yet the small firms are in as great a need of this skill.

UNITY OF COMMAND

To emphasise the importance yet the difficulties of line management the following quotation from Luther Gulick is relevant:

"From the earliest times it has been recognised that nothing but confusion arises under multiple command. 'A man cannot serve two masters' was a theological argument because it was accepted as a principle of human relations in everyday life. In administration this is known as the principle of 'unity of command'. The principle may be stated as follows:

"A workman subject to orders from several superiors will be

confused, a workman subject to orders from but one superior may be methodical, efficient and responsible. Unit of command thus refers to those who are commanded, not to those who issue commands.

"The significance of this principle in the process of co-ordination must not be lost sight of. In building a structure of co-ordination it is often tempting to set up more than one boss for a man who is doing work which has more than one relationship. Even as great a philosopher of management as Taylor fell into this error in setting up separate foreman to deal with machinery, with materials, with speed, etc., each with the power of giving orders directly to the individual workman. The rigid adherence to the principle of unity of command may have its absurdities: these are, however, unimportant in comparison with the certainty of confusion, inefficiency and irresponsibility which arise from the violation of the principle."

The importance of providing the opportunity for people to understand and take on the duties of management early in their career is insufficiently appreciated, particularly among highly specialised technical staff. Yet if these principles are not woven into the fabric of technical and administrative responsibility, the problems we are seeing today will greatly multiply. Technology must be tempered by responsibility.

THE DULLNESS OF THE WORKING DAY

By 1847 the length of the working day, up to sixteen hours for children and adults, had become a major issue, leading to the passing of the "Ten Hours Bill": 130 years later the appropriateness of an eight-hour working day is being brought into question for different but cogent reasons: many working men and women are now condemned to unrelieved boredom in contrast to the physical exhaustion of their predecessors. Variety is so much a part of a doctor's life and so valuable in creating its spice and satisfaction that perhaps he takes it for granted in the lives of others: yet the evidence is clear that as we "educate" people to even higher "standards" there is a failure to provide them with the equivalent challenge which leads to contentment.

The reshaping of industrial relations must come and it will do so more quickly when men and women are given the opportunity to express themselves, to vary their activities, and to feel that in the job they do they can recognise a meaningful relationship to the end product. The doctor in industry can assist in its reshaping. This means that he must first understand the problems, then appreciate in what capacity he can assist. Very often this may be done in the simplest of ways, by easing communication between the worker and his management. The general practitioner's worker-patient more than once in his career will be involved in an all too common and poorly managed altercation with his bosses, with the inevitable outcome of resentment. This can often be dissipated by talking it over with someone: that someone could be his doctor, for a somatic symptom may disguise a neurosis brought on by frustration. Obviously no doctor can spare the time to investigate this aspect of the life of every patient he sees, but awareness of the possibility will alert him – people express their problems in many different ways, as this case report illustrates:

P.A.B., a 55-year-old works manager of a precision engineering firm, came to the clinic complaining of hoarseness which had recurred every two or three months for the past year. He had been to his general practitioner who had examined him and referred him for a specialist opinion: the specialist had reassured him that there was nothing to find and in particular had excluded cancer, which had been a niggling worry to P.A.B. The industrial physician who saw him remarked a thick-set, voluble, rather plethoric Yorkshire-man who smoked cigarettes heavily. He was a likeable character and proved willing to discuss his whole life situation. But first an examination was repeated to exclude obvious local disease.

The picture of this man's problem began to emerge quite early in the discussion; a man who had never lost a day's work through illness, whose relations with his employees were forthright but flexible and he had avoided any major problems. Until recently morale at the works, among some one hundred men, had been good, but lately there had been a walk-out, the cause of which he had found difficult to identify. His personal life presented no obvious clue: his children, two daughters, were both happily married. He and his wife were very attached to each other but he admitted that she was somewhat rigid in her acceptance of slight deviations from her code of behaviour, one of these being temperance with alcohol. This had never reared its head until the past year, when P.A.B. had found himself stopping off for a few drinks, mostly beer, after work, on his way home. The reason for this was that he had begun to find the need to relieve his frustration built up during the working day over the behaviour of his co-director, who handled all administration and accounts. This man, older than P.A.B. by ten years, was incapable of taking the responsibility given to him by the directors of the parent company in another city: he had developed the habit of a prolonged lunch "hour" of nearly three hours, returning in a condition which matched his alcohol consumption, after which he was useless for the rest of the day, leaving much of the responsibility on P.A.B.'s shoulders. He had managed to conceal his habits from the parent company directors and P.A.B. could not bring himself to tell them directly. It was then that his hoarseness and sometimes complete loss of voice began to affect him.

When it was pointed out to him that this symptom resulted from his frustration through loyalty on the one hand, and on the other a desperate need to confide in someone, he accepted this explanation of his otherwise unexplainable complaint – i.e. that he was preventing himself saying what needed to be said. Furthermore, when the physician found a means to let the other directors know and see for themselves the condition of P.A.B.'s colleague, they were able to resolve the problem by the latter's retirement: P.A.B. had no further trouble either with his voice or his wife! The men on the shop floor, who had realised the way things were going, were able to give their loyalty once again to the firm and the episode was closed.

THE INDUSTRIAL PHYSICIAN

The body and spirit of an industry can be just as individual, with its idiosyncrasies and susceptibilities, as those of one of its employees; this may not be sufficiently appreciated. Here an independent interpreter, the industrial physician, can be useful, but he should not set himself up as a judge in so far as his actions might be so interpreted by others. The channels by which he can achieve firm *rapport* with management are seldom obvious or even available and may have to be created, sometimes with considerable difficulty. The place in the organisation where the physician may be said to identify himself and the line of management through which he functions remain subject to the circumstances of every individual appointment. Unless there is some overwhelming reason, the industrial physician, full- or part-time, should have direct access to the overall manager, with the mundane items of his day-to-day counsels being actioned at a lower level of authority. This may be seen to appear to contradict the statement earlier about the "unity of command". This emphasises the need for a definitive policy on the executive action that should be taken, *not by the doctor but by the administration*. The managing director should not be hampered with daily trivia, but on the other hand neither should he be deprived of advice which can assist him in his overall policy making. The doctor should therefore advise directly all unit managers in affairs relating to their departments: when necessary he should inform the chief of those circumstances which require his action or of which he should be aware. The judge of when to do this must be the doctor, who decides whether the unit manager should also be involved: there can be very few occasions when he should not, and the damage that can be done by thoughtlessly going over his head can be devastating and irreparable. The role of the doctor is advisory, not executive – apart from his own professional unit – and thus the principle of "unity of command" is not strained in his counselling of management. Nevertheless, the principle should always be in his mind, because people are understandably sensitive; offence can easily be taken when none is intended. One of the most frustrating problems is when distorted information gives rise to alarm, anxiety and non-co-operation. It takes a steady nerve to deal with this sequence, to quietly sort out the tangle and soothe people's feelings.

DOCTORS AND MANAGERS

Doctors are sometimes reproached for having a detached and high-minded Grundyism when discussing with non-medical and non-professional people the purpose and content of commerce. The latter is principally to make profits, he is told, and the industry isn't there for the benefit of the employees. Looked at in terms of single enterprises this may have some logic in it, but over the country as a whole commerce and industry are there for the benefit of employees, for we are all employees and consumers at the same time. This sort of argument can very easily create a wide gulf between management and medical adviser unless the latter is aware of the danger, and prepared to concede that the other may have a point. The art of compromise is a necessary, more than just a useful, component of the industrial physician's stock-in-trade. It is to be regretted that despite the prolonged training undertaken by young doctors, few during their course have had presented to them, in a systematic manner, the problems of people at work. The opportunity to become aware that even in their personal experiences of hospital and clinic, the same human interactions occur and need to be recognised, contained and managed, is governed only by their own perceptiveness and sensibility. The medical student is taught how to manage a sick person with disease, but this is limited to the duration of the dialogue between them and the subsequent technical discussion of the patient's care: as soon as the dialogue is over, the management of the patient passes to the doctor's assistants, the nurses, social workers and others. Apart from consulting and occasional guidance, the doctor may not have any management responsibility towards non-professional staff. But in relation to his own professional organisation, management does arise and is now recognised by the provision of training to doctors in the hospital and local health services.

The non-doctor manager cannot limit his involvement with his working group – he is paid to become continuously involved and to manage individuals and groups of apparently healthy persons throughout his working day; his only retreat, like that of the union-organised worker, is by the withdrawal of his labour. Up until recently this has not been through strike action or short-term illness: it has had either to be by resignation or following physical or mental breakdown after a prolonged period of stress. The extent, quality and effects of stress in himself or in others are not always recognised by the manager, unless he has been specifically trained to do so. It is one of the responsibilities of the doctor in industry to be on the look out for this contingency and take action before serious illness is precipitated. The ramifications which may accompany the careful investigations in such a case can be as fascinating and frustrating as those encountered during the unravelling of a serious organic disease, but with the additional spice that the organisation must be held together, continue to operate and be productive meanwhile.

The physician should come to feel that he is a part of the business undertaking: he must avoid being handed responsibility which is rightly that of executive management and he must preserve and stimulate management's awareness of its own social responsibility. The doctor's role may sometimes sharpen that awareness to the point of creating new problems, but at the same time the doctor may help to lighten management's load. He should always be ready to listen, the quintessence of the art of medicine. The support of management is a primary role shared equally with a personal responsibility to each employee, but with complete respect for the confidence of the individual.

5 Human Behaviour in Industry or Industrial Psychology

Some words of Sir Frank Fraser Darling are taken from a penetrating and thought-provoking address in a symposium on the problems of world medicine. Its author expressed the view that disease diatheses or tendencies are possessed by most of us, waiting only for the right inducement before leaping into activity or beginning an insidious erosion of the body's defences. We now know the nature of a few of these mechanisms: some are psychological, of which grief is a not uncommon example; others can be chemical, among which the carcinogens or cancer-provoking agents have gained a leading place in our attention; and yet others may be physical. The speaker emphasised the effect of psychological infectiousness acting upon a susceptible population, exhibiting certain of the characteristics of micro-organisms, notably the increase in virulence the greater the number of susceptible victims.

"Our friend Humphrey Osmond directed our attention to late eighteenth and early nineteenth century mental hospitals run by Quakers and similarly-minded men: it seems that the degree of privacy available to each patient, small groupings of between four and ten, and walks in surroundings of natural foliage had marked curative effects. Planning and architecture were important as well as the personalities of the doctors and attendants. If amelioration of environmental stress can have such a marked effect in a community of the mentally sick, we should be ready to analyse and understand it much better in the so-called sane, larger community which mentally desires to resist stress and not succumb to it, but which in fact does considerably succumb in obscure psychosomatic diseases, in syndromes of violence and mass hysteria."

To those working among industrial populations the relevance of these remarks will not be lost, for they have observed the disruptions which seem so common in large industries contrasted with the relative freedom of dislocation of work among smaller coteries. Therefore it will be useful to review the social forces acting within a manufacturing or servicing industry, a large or small office community or even in a hospital environment.

First is the vital reason for which the industrial organisation exists: the extent to which this is understood by the employees and the knowledge they possess of the success or frustrations of the enterprise. Next comes the nature and quality of the administrative structure which identifies the lines of responsibility, decision making and communications. Finally, but not the least important, are the motivations of the human power-houses which provide the energy and expertise: these must be co-ordinated towards a well-defined goal and for which everybody in the organisation should have a respect and a pride. This may sound a naïve and idealistic picture of an industrial enterprise, but such organisations do exist, to provide the examples of the basis upon which people should be able to work satisfyingly together. The traditional picture which we possess of the village crafts and other local enterprises largely satisfied these criteria, and explained their success in creating local industrial harmony over many centuries until the advent of mechanisation.

With the rapid change in the pattern of work following the introduction of mechanical power in the eighteenth century, men began to lose both their identity as craftsmen and the knowledge of the goal to which they worked, for this was now being set by others than themselves who were remote and often unknown. Thus slowly did the pattern of industrial psychological maladies of our time begin to form, much of it associated with stress, resentment, frustration and boredom.

Doctors should be concerned with people rather than profits; those in charge of industry should be concerned with both equally. Industrial psychology is the understanding of the behaviour of people at work in the restricted sense of being in gainful employment in industry, itself a subculture of our total environment. In this subculture there is expressed great individuality, dependent upon physical and psychological maturity but conditioned also by factors outside a person's control. The worker must respond to these conditions and come to terms with them. A huge network of human relationships may be discerned in which the behaviour of any one worker must be judged against the background of the culture from which he comes: this may either potentiate or conflict with the

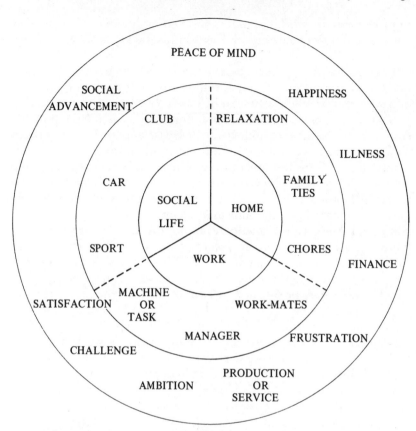

Fig. 6 Working man and his whole-life experience: he is at the centre of his universe, but the boundaries can become blurred and the relationship realigned.

atmosphere in which he now finds himself. His successful integration will depend upon his maturity and adaptability coupled with the recognition he receives for the effort he makes. This aspect of the background culture is very important. In this country many older workers recall the manner of living in which they grew up: the unemployment and insecurity of their parents' lives, yet strengthened by loyalties and articles of faith whether by religious or other strong local ties. The younger worker today has been exposed to the permissive egalitarian material culture of post-war years: has tasted the pleasures of possessions and felt the very human urge to satisfy his appetite for more. The pace and strength of this demand for personal wealth have outstripped the more traditional sentiment of being satisfied with one's lot, providing the conditions of work are acceptable. This philosophy is decreasingly effective despite the continued

improvement in working conditions and provisions made to cope
with sudden loss of earnings through injury, sickness or redundancy.

Beneath the veneer of this driving, thrusting materialistic urge
lies the outstandingly important desire to identify and be identified,
not necessarily as an individual but as a member of an organisation
of people to which a loyalty can be given. In earlier times the family
occupied this position; with the break-up of the extended family life,
still seen in rural and undeveloped areas, and owing to physical
separation and educational and cultural chasms, the worker's
loyalty has perhaps become centred in his small occupational group.
This would possibly show the strongest organisation and give him
the moral support he needs. Man is a sociable and naturally gre-
garious animal; it is this informal occupational group which may
command his greatest loyalty even to the embarrassment of his
family: we have seen this in recent unofficial strikes where union-
financed support has been withheld. This loyalty creates identity,
the one potentiating the other. The urge or craving for identity which
we all possess may be satisfied early in life as with the child born into
a family rich in simple culture and faith: he will mature to use what
education is given him in steadily progressive steps towards responsibility and enjoy the satisfaction arising from his work and social
activities. Identity provides status, function, security and social
responsibility: in these days of angry discontent the search for identity
may lead to the antithesis, social irresponsibility or what seems
to be so in the eyes of conservative citizens. It is when the powerful
biological machine is presented with an impatient psychological
ferment, the product of immaturity and intellectual precocity, that
an explosive mixture is compounded.

The need for status is basic and together with the desire for
prestige should not be brushed aside: it should be accepted, moulded
and co-ordinated. Without status people will not be effective; with it
they will learn to work together productively. This leads naturally
to function which is the sharing in the life and activity of the group in
a purposeful manner, creating a sense of dependency within it and
adhering to the rules of procedure even though these are seldom
expressed. The man who works too fast creates a jarring note which
upsets the rhythm of output and the mental composure of those at
work with him. But once the functional niche has been gained and
consolidated, a feeling of security must follow. It is, however, in the
doctor's consulting room that the effects of the struggles to reach
these goals are seen, among those who have suffered their problems
and failures in comparative silence and in doing so have destroyed
their poise and confidence; yet many of these people may have
achieved "success". Perhaps nowhere is this better illustrated than

in the universities: while the student health physicians are helping those who silently struggle, the proctors and police cope with the rebels expressing their inability, and often incapacity to function and identify, claiming that social responsibility is denied to them. The character and competence of a working group will often determine the individual's behaviour, a phenomenon sometimes used for the rehabilitation of some of society's young malefactors and other ill-adjusted people. It is interesting to observe the behaviour of people when in different company: in the industrial context this is shown by the variation in productive output.

A word about working numbers. Groups of between five and ten people have been found most suitable by long practice and confirmed by industrial psychologists: this restricted figure allows a person to relate to others and find a niche. The size of a factory, on the other hand, is more difficult to decide upon, but there is good evidence that it is not easy to infuse a sense of responsibility into units greater than 500. The number crops up again when considering the size of hospitals, military formations and other organisations. Experience has taught people that, beyond a certain figure, a sense of personal involvement evaporates and responsibility is then left to those relatively apart, either in the union or management: the opportunity for shared responsibility throughout the plant progressively declines.

A recent letter in the national press from a Southampton University student has drawn attention to similar experience in a social milieu: ". . . In those days 'student bodies' were far smaller, and this, I think, is the key to the present malaise. Though most students today – repeat 'most' – are potentially positive citizens, their trust and interest in each other (and in society at large) begin to disintegrate when they are lumped together in thousands. We reckoned that a 'student body' could remain integrated and lively as long as its membership was about 250. Its saturation point was 300. . . . Therefore, if there must be 'industrial legislation' let one simple law be put to the aid of students: that each local 'body' should contain an absolute maximum of 300 members, each independent with its own council, life and finances. This would build a cohesive cellular structure in the country, it would make the National Union of Students more mobile and representative, it would limit the dangers of misspent public monies and it would give fresh heart to many students who feel that they are victims of an increasingly 'depressed industry'."

Most industrial psychologists agree that the happiness and efficiency of people at work is less dependent on their physical environmental conditions than on the subjective sense of their own usefulness and significance. This is perhaps why the production records of small firms, often with substandard working conditions and housekeeping, stand up to and exceed those of the potentially more efficient large industrial complexes. The man (or woman) in a small factory means something to the boss: his (or her) absence often creates a major hiatus and he (or she) can feel appreciated and useful. But this element of absenteeism, while not necessarily having a direct medical bearing, may enable the doctor to see the results of some of his population's failure to achieve a challenge and satisfaction at their job. If it would benefit his patient, he should be in a position to interpret this to management. Every day more of our neighbours and patients are becoming increasingly bored with their daily existence under this tyranny of automation and anonymity. The result can be escape into mental and physical fatigue or violent reaction, now being used by unfriendly elements to foment disruption of our industrial potential. If we extrapolate these views we will be entering the field of politics and industrial relations, both beyond our present brief, yet I would like to quote from John Bosworth, percipient recorder of the industrial scene in the national press: "Nor is there any security of compensation in close contact with other work people. Mechanisation which earlier decimated the officers is now cutting swathes through the other ranks. Even in the pits, where the tradition of working comradeship is at its strongest, mechanisation has pushed men so far apart on some jobs that they have to be brought back into contact with closed circuit television."

I have aimed to show you the character of some of the psychological disorders engendered by adverse environmental conditions acting upon people at work. I do not say that these effects all stem from work, for the interactions within a person's whole life experience must ruffle his equanimity from time to time. The remarkable thing is that, just as with infectious disease, so many people escape major consequences. By understanding the natural history of these disorders the doctor can relate his patient's problems earlier and have means to alleviate them. This predicates a partnership, even if this is loose and occasional, with management at all its levels. For this partnership to exist, some form of bridge must be constructed between the general practitioner and industry. One of the main components of this bridge is a common appreciation by management and doctors of the human problems which touch upon one another's work. These involve the design of work which should avoid, as far as possible, having to adapt the man to the job but rather fit the job to the man. The selection of people, the ability to predict their attitudes to work and specific jobs; the provision of good training; a proper staff structure and promotion prospects to satisfy ambition and recognise talent; the need to appreciate the importance and difficulty of separating frustration due to these causes from the plain discontent of a boring and unsatisfying job. The closer some people approach their goal, real or imaginary, the more frustrated and discontented they may become, a psychological inverse square law for those who have set themselves too high a target.

Another basic element for bridge building is the recognition of the effects upon sick and injured workmen of prolonged absence from work and the almost equally important consequences on their work-mates and management. All three – worker, doctor and management – may be partially or wholly to blame for the situations which do arise. The worker who is playing on the apparent benefits of sickness absence; the doctor who is ignorant of his patient's potential and conditions of work, and the manager who doesn't want him back until he is 100 per cent fit. Short-term absences for "sickness" are increasing at a greater frequency then the length of sickness spells, which suggests that on the whole the worker does not like to upset his social relationships at work beyond a point of no return, for this would mean discarding his workmates and losing his identity: we see this too often as the lot of retired people. Despite or because of his own long history of mental instability, William Cowper, in his poem "Retirement", did very wisely lament that

> "Absence of Occupation is not rest
> A mind quite vacant is a mind distressed."

Return to work should be as early as feasible, and it is here that doctors and other medical workers may need to take issue with industrialists, who may see no profit in the short term by taking in a partially disabled worker to do a job at a slower pace or perhaps to do one that doesn't need doing. Selective Employment Tax has not helped managers to overcome their prejudice. In the long term the benefits of early rehabilitation can be lasting to patient and those among whom he works. Many firms today will facilitate an early return to work even to the extent of transporting workers to and from their homes. More government help, direct or indirect, might be given to industry to encourage this practice.

Increased absenteeism among women workers has been referred to in a previous chapter; there is no evidence of a heightened dis-position to occupational diseases, but the biological differences of man and woman do account for the frequency to some extent. Probably variations in motivation are most influential, springing as they do from biological and environmental stresses whether domestic or at work. The value of female occupational health nursing contact with women workers and their supervisors cannot be over-emphasised. It is practicable to give support to both psycho-neurotic and somatically ill patients in the working environment, and this aspect of occupational health nursing can be compared in importance to the help and support of businessman may need in his financial situation from his consultants and his bankers. A married woman worker has to manage her divided responsibilities: the strain of trying to do this, or indeed the failure, may lead her to escape into illness and absenteeism: when this happens a social and occupational history is mandatory when attempting to help her.

Much has been written on the subject of industrial psychology: but when all is said and done on the lines we have discussed, it is the individual worker as a thinking person who is the matrix of the problem. It is his preparation for life which really matters, for his reaction to conditions at work will be governed by the sort of person he is. Nothing therefore could be more important than that young people should be given the opportunity of learning about themselves, their social relations with others and how to bear responsibility, together with the long-term benefits of rising to the challenge.

6 Industrial Relations and "Work Systems"

More people are becoming employed by large organisations, some closely integrated and possessing a well-developed and widely-embracing occupational health service; others have come together in loose-knit commercial groups as a result of take-over policies and amalgamations. Members of this latter group often consist of many small industrial units left to get along on their own to make a profit – if they don't, then they are shut down or sold and there may be little chance of the employees obtaining continuing employment within the parent organisation in the same area. Most of these smaller units do not have an occupational health service, but by the same token neither does the possession of an occupational health service *per se* give the firm any specific advantage in profit-making, although it may mean that management has some understanding of the less clearly defined problems of their employees: only in the long run may this appreciation reveal itself in better and more sustained production. It may also suggest that other aspects of industrial relations are on a better footing, although it would be an unwise assumption because of the many other external influences involved. It is a sad reflection of the attitude of a competitive society that when the economic wind blows cold the victims are very often those activities which do not clearly and at once declare a cash benefit: the first among these may be the occupational health service and other social–welfare activities which are greatly needed to place our industrial environment on a healthy footing. Unless or until the benefits of such services, assuming these can be separately identified in our welfare society today, are seen to relate to the individual industrial economy, this situation will continue. The fact is that the organisation and operating cost of assessing the value of these services is generally unacceptable to a firm's accountants: they will deny that benefits from an outlay such as redeveloping the administration to control excessive sickness wastage may give a realistic return. One of the strongest arguments, for which there is some validity, is that even when given healthy conditions of work there are still many other background factors both within and outside the control of industry itself which are influencing the one identifiable health statistic by which productivity can be gauged; that is the sickness absence rate. It must be remembered that both sickness and accident absence remove the individual from the work situation: this may be fortuitous or as a result of factors engineered by the individual or his work environment. Nevertheless, it is worth reviewing the research that has been done on more general lines because there are many managers and employees today who do have respect for each other and for whom this information can serve as a guide in reframing their present and future approach to working conditions. Earlier I have presented a picture of the behaviour of people at work: this is the key to the understanding of all industrial relations for it must impinge on and result from people's prejudices, tolerances and will to work.

Whereas the study of toxic properties of industrial materials and physical conditions at work have been the preoccupation of industrial medicine over the last 100 years, today mental health must take precedence in line with the situation in community medicine. Those added factors, outside an individual's domestic and familial circle, his industrial organisation, the environment, the working group, racial integration, the promotion ladder, and its antithesis the demotion and redundancy fear, must now be accepted as relevant. Competition with its challenge and disappointment; the frustrations, some related to the personality of the worker, others to the inherent nature of the job, such as the insignificance of the action; repetitiveness or the boredom of automation, all of these are now the subject of intense research in this country and abroad. It is worth emphasising, at the risk of repetition, that a work environment in which these can operate is not limited to industrial enterprises but embraces all those organisations who supply a need, provide a service for clientele – what are called service industries – who manufacture a commodity such as water or electricity, or run a transportation or communications system. They must therefore include schools, colleges, hospitals, laboratories and a host of smaller "you name it" organisations. With the increasing distance today between work and home, the domestic and community social factors which once allowed for some elasticity in the worker's output or absence no longer are appreciated by his boss or even his work-mates; he is on his own, he has to find his own remedies to situations he faces or quickly adopt those of the working group, *force majeure*. This may not be satisfactory for everyone, but it is the system, and if a worker goes against the system, whether it be of management, unions or his close working group, he has to stand the chance of being penalised.

At the basis of our understanding of a person at work should be the happiness which he (or she) experiences both on and from the job he is doing; the historical and traditional association of work with suffering stems, in the main, from the exposures in the nineteenth century of the social ills of the Industrial Revolution. For most people today the physical suffering has been removed only to be replaced by mental disturbance, often of insidious onset and which may finally be expressed by aggressive reaction, withdrawal, psychosomatic illness, or frank mental breakdown. If it is accepted that work is necessary for sustained happiness and health over and above the social obligation to work which is generally honoured in our present conventions of culture, then it must be made to appear so; too often today this is not the case. With modern refinements of technique and engineering we are beginning to move from the era of actual physical quantity of effort to the newer concept of an acceptable quality in the nature of work, when the real time required to do the work may be embarrassingly short. We see this reduction in worktime on the shop floor as a result of both the newer techniques and the unions' demands, and the concept of short-time has become part of our daily thinking and, for many, living. Here lies the potential danger, for the increasing periods of leisure may themselves foment a sense of unfulfilment with insufficient gratification unless people can be introduced to the idea of using their time constructively in the widest sense: this will require some re-education. The expression of dissatisfaction with the nature of the work is related to intelligence, education and personal preference, not all of which may be present or acting together: with the gradual but steady improvement of the national educational level, we might expect more not less dissatisfaction unless jobs are redesigned to meet this eventuality. There is an inverse relationship between the acceptance of drudgery and level of education.

A knowledge of human relations is not the prerogative of doctors, psychologists or social workers. Considerable expertise is possessed by all levels of management within industry, although there are still wide gaps and notable failures. Management and trades unions, both on the shop floor and at high levels, do practise human relations successfully, but this is seldom of news value; nevertheless, throughout industry there are many daily examples of the truth of this.

Any approach to occupational health, including mental health, should be a partnership between management, unions and employees; at present an occupational health service to many workers has still a paternalistic flavour because it is financed by the management – this will continue to happen in this country until the employees and their unions become convinced of the value of such services, and press their case to achieve a shared responsibility. Government action could catalyse this by bringing all groups together, removing mutual suspicion and creating a firm partnership. Rather than direct legislation, indirect encouragement by preferential tax benefits to those organisations and individuals following its advice would seem the wisest approach. At the present time it is imperative, if we are to see a widening of the occupational health services of this country, that managers should be made more aware of how the human problems arise and their frequent consequence, the generation of neuroses on the shop floors and in the offices. These can be prevented, alleviated and sometimes cured by timely recognition, and sympathetic and confident handling, not always necessitating referral to a doctor. Unfortunately an understanding of occupational health services in management education is still not sufficiently appreciated by either the organisers or participants. The motivations of security, competition, self-esteem, gratification, and sense of contribution, among many others, which are today behind the will to work are at once the cause of some people's success but many people's inability to achieve stability and lead to their subsequent neurotic behaviour. At the same time personal responsibility stands in danger of being eroded by social welfare programmes which remove the necessary stimulus to work from those people just on the borderline of social irresponsibility. You may initially remove or lessen the causes of neurosis by ill-designed or unwisely directed social welfare only to replace them with the still socially unacceptable stigmata directed to those not working: these are generated within a tax-paying community by the current ethos of working to earn one's living.

The effect of shift systems upon a worker's health has long been a bone of contention among people having to undergo shiftwork and those organising shift systems. Basically it can be said that if the worker can see a good reason for being on shift, either permanently or at intervals, he will accept it with the qualifications inherent in the possible disruption of his domestic and social life. No convincing studies have ever shown shift systems *per se* to be injurious: they are apparently necessary; they continue and are, in the main accepted. There is a strong possibility that in the future, to adjust to business and social pressures of various kinds, their need will increase to cover a larger section of the population. At the present time it is estimated that there are about one million people on permanent or temporary shift duties. In factories women generally do not undertake shift duties unless certain conditions are fulfilled, and then only with the agreement of the Factory Inspectorate. Yet women have undertaken shift work for many years in the service industries such as hospitals and communications systems without any identifiable ill-effect. Research only confirms this, but nothing can alter the fact that some people either cannot or will not adapt to the alteration in their social and biological cycle. This decision as to whether to continue shift work should be their's alone, even if it means changing jobs. Nevertheless, employment agreements usually contain provisions for some form of shift work and choice of job is therefore limited.

Physiological circadian rhythms: circa diem, about a day: man's adaptability, more successful than that of other animals, has governed the nature of his evolution – we still may see evidence of this in the sequence of developmental changes taking place in the fertilised human ovum in the pregnant uterus. These changes tell us the story of human evolution from a single-celled organism through the stage of the gill-breathing fish to final dependence upon lung respiration needed when our ancestors moved out of the sea to live permanently on dry land. Chemical changes in his tissue fluids also occurred, evidence of which persists today. The stimulus to his adaptive mechanisms derives from the environment, itself basically dependent on the passage of the earth round the sun, with consequent day and night and attendant temperature changes. A more recent human development has been the assumption of a crop-gathering and animal husbandry pattern of food production requiring it to be taken at regular intervals in contrast to the wild food gatherer who ate as he gathered or the hunter who ate only when he killed, which might mean at intervals of some days. Examples of these ways of life still exist in primitive communities, among the bushmen of Africa and the aboriginals of Australia. More enlightened folk who still live by hunting, the Eskimos being the outstanding example, have learnt to store their food and have developed more regular eating habits. We have become people of habit, with rigid social customs, variations of which may be seen in every community on every island and continent. Chief among these habits are sleeping, eating and defaecation or bowel opening: individuals vary greatly in their response to the need to adjust these basic habits to meet a changing requirement.

The timing of the body's metabolic routine, outwardly shown by

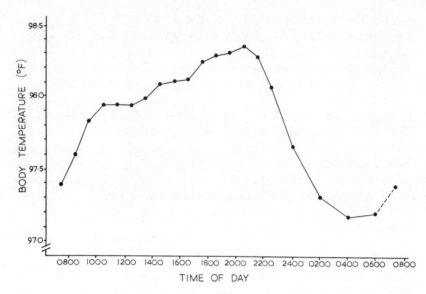

Fig. 7 Two-point rolling mean body temperatures of 59 subjects at 20 times of day (average of two trials). Body temperature rhythm over a 24-hour period. (*From W. P. Colquhoun, M. J. F. Blake and R. S. Edwards "Experimental Studies in Shift-work". Ergonomics, Vol. 11, 437–453, 1968.*)

these basic functions, is governed by an intricate system of feed-back mechanisms involving principally nervous, hormone, enzyme and blood systems, all of which are closely integrated functionally. Any disturbance of this integration, in effect a careful habitual balance, will induce a lag or debt before the system can accommodate to the new demands. Some people are able to readjust quickly and soon overcome this lag, others do so more slowly and some have the greatest difficulty. The metabolic function of the body may be crudely but honestly measured by the body temperature: this is known to vary as much as $2°F$ ($1·111°C$) during the twenty-four hours. During the hours of greatest activity for people working during the day, from the time of getting up to mid-afternoon, the body temperature rises slowly. As food is taken in and burnt in the process of muscle activity and the other metabolic chemical reactions, the body heat increases as more is produced than can be lost during the same period. If heat loss is too rapid, as for instance by men working insufficiently clad doing little physical work, such as a fork-lift operator in a meat cold store or by young hikers sheltering from wind and rain in the hills, then a feed-back mechanism would at once operate to quicken their metabolic rate and muscle activity; the resulting shivering, which increases metabolism by sustained muscle activity produces further internal heat to maintain normal body temperature. If this mechanism fails, as it may during sickness, in old age or under the influence of some drugs, the body temperature will fall and the activity of the body will be reduced. Such a sequence will occur in *all* animals, whether warm- or cold-blooded, and is easily seen in the latter by the varying activity of insects, reptiles and fish during hot and cold weather. But mammalian, marsupial and avian animals are potentially capable of resisting this process of cooling or overheating and the intricate and delicate system which does this is known as the homeostatic mechanism. By these criteria we can understand how, towards the end of a working day, bodily efficiency gradually weakens; it will temporarily recover after the evening meal only to lessen again, together with body temperature, until, in the fastness of the night at about four o'clock in the morning it reaches its lowest point coinciding with deepest sleep. This cycle comes closest to the hibernation experienced by some warm-blooded animals in response to an unfriendly, cold external environment. Thus it seems reasonable not to require people to be on their toes at four a.m. unless they have become fully adapted to the changed time for their maximum output. This adaptation can come about relatively quickly provided there is no mental resistance and provided the work being done is both interesting and demanding, mentally or physically. Thus it is that airline pilots are able to adjust to the irregular requirements of their job: on the other hand, simple repetitive work may be accompanied by an increased frequency of minor accidents due to inattention and fatigue. People finding difficulty in adjusting may complain of or be more sensitive to general bodily and nervous disorders, respiratory and gastro-intestinal upsets, headaches, dizziness and a host of minor, ill-defined symptoms.

While I have described the adjustment of the circadian or twenty-four hour rhythm in the shift worker, the same mechanism requires to be considered by those flying through the different time-zones either in an east to west or west to east direction. The wisdom of whether a business executive, professional man or a politician should enter into important decisional discussions immediately upon arrival perhaps at a point in his twenty-four hour rhythm corresponding to the time of his lowest metabolic activity (four a.m.) is, to say the least, questionable. This should be self-evident, yet is done every day by countless travellers. Investigations have shown that these people do feel the effect upon their sleep, bowels and eating habits; even so 30 per cent of business executives in one study conducted negotiations immediately on arrival, and a further 20 per cent within twelve hours of arrival. Thus a total of 50 per cent did so

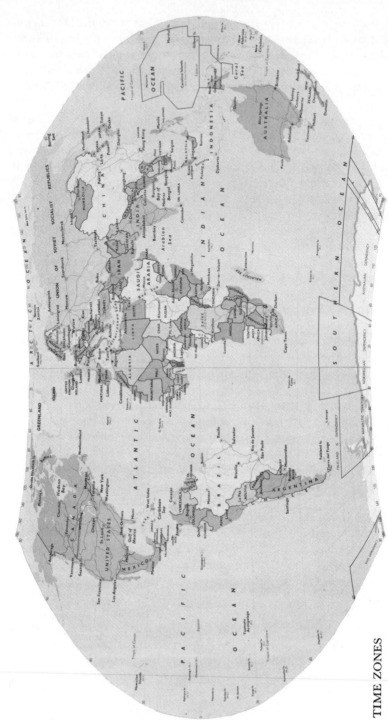

TIME ZONES

Time changes by one hour for every fifteen meridians of longitude. For example, Greenwich is at 0°: Fiji is at 180°: there is thus twelve hours time difference.   (*Acknowledgment to George Philip and Son, Ltd.*)

before going to bed, despite the fact that over 80 per cent claimed that they needed a night's sleep before being fully fit. So you will see that there is still a big educational breakthrough to be made. Advice to a person making transatlantic or other long (five or more time zones) east–west and west–east journeys should be given as follows:

(a) A flight should be chosen so that where possible the subject arrives shortly before his usual bedtime.
(b) On arrival the subject should go to his hotel and soon afterwards go to bed, having at least one worthwhile sleep period before entering into business negotiations.
(c) These should, therefore, not be commenced until the day after arrival if at all possible.
(d) If, however, it is essential to hold a conference soon after arrival, then the conference should be held at a time when the subject would normally be awake in his home environment.

It is most undesirable for business to be conducted when the executive would normally, in his home environment, be asleep. He may imagine that he is up to his usual standard of acumen and efficiency and, like an alcoholic, be quite euphoric about it. Objective analysis, however, reveals a marked falling off in performance under such circumstances.

(e) On return to his home country, although an immediate report may be made, the writing of final reports should be delayed for at least twenty-four to forty-eight hours until the subject has had an opportunity to readapt.

The stresses resulting from shift work and rapid air travel are most liable to disturb those body functions which are generally regarded as the basic determinants of a healthy state–sleep, eating and regular bowel action. There is no longer any dispute that workers on rotating night shift do not obtain as much actual sleep as their colleagues on day work, but providing the shift cycle is relatively short, any sleep debt which may accrue should be resolved during subsequent sleep periods of day shift. Thus it is the type of shift cycle and its accompanying rest periods which control the general subjective feeling of well-being by the worker: the more frequent the change the less chance of sleep debt building up: despite this many workers are of the erroneous opinion that rapid cycle changes are bad for the health. Much the same can be said about the effect of shift work on appetite and enjoyment of food: both sleep and eating are relevant to a person's susceptibility to neurosis. No evidence exists that, by itself, shift work is a cause of gastro-intestinal disease, but undoubtedly certain individuals may be more prone to develop symptoms than others, and among them are those who already have a history of peptic ulcer. One situation which must be carefully considered is that of the diabetic worker. If he or she is not taking insulin, then no real problem need arise, but when insulin is required to control the diabetic state dosage is designed to cater for steady state activity and balanced food intake, it is obviously unrealistic for such a diabetic worker to undergo frequent changes of work shift and have to continually adjust meal times, meal quantity and the quality and dose of the insulin. This individual should restrict his work to permanent day or night work and not require his diminished reserve of liver and pancreatic function to cope with the surges of demand which cannot be met rapidly. The treatment of diabetes rests principally upon the establishment of habit; the physiological functions of the body come to depend on this; remember that the diabetic's adaptive capacity is more brittle than a normal person's.

Alteration in bowel function, in our present context more usually constipation, is due to interference with habit: it is both a possibility and for those going on shift for the first time a probability unless they take care to spend time and trouble to avoid it. It amounts to no more hazard than the interference with the bowels which happens on holiday; shift duties may be considered an indirect cause. No serious consequences have ever been reported; provided people take the trouble to see that the bowels have time to open, they will usually do so: the post-meal toilet session is the corner-stone of good bowel habits.

General physical and mental health is dependent upon many factors other than the work situation; some people on permanent rotating shift duties are self-selected and have found, for various reasons, that they maintain better health by so doing. These reasons may vary from food habits, nature of a permanent night job with relatively few workers and an added degree of responsibility. Social reasons relate to attitudes of wife and children, and financial benefit. It is interesting that in this self-selected group of shift workers such effects as lowered sickness absence rates and greater longevity after retirement have been observed; the secret seems to lie in the element of choice which these people make in their manner of life and work. But where choice does not operate then the neurotic dispositions, which we all possess to a greater or lesser extent come into play, their effect depending upon the degree of disturbance to our way of of life.

Having generalised to affirm that shift work is harmless, we should again emphasise that there are those who may not be suited, such as the worker with a peptic ulcer, the diabetic on insulin treatment,

A SAMPLE ROTATING SHIFT SCHEDULE

Days of the week

Hours working	M	T	W	T	F	S	S	M	T	W	T	F	S	S	M	T	W	T	F	S	S
7.00 a.m. – 3.00 p.m.	A*	D	D	A	A	B	B	B	A	A	B	B	C	C	C	B	B	C	C	D	D
3.00 p.m. – 11.00 p.m.	B	B	B	C	C	D	D	C	C	C	D	D	A	A	D	D	D	A	A	B	B
11.00 p.m. – 7.00 a.m.	C	C	C	D	D	A	A	D	D	D	A	A	B	B	A	A	A	B	B	C	C

* The letters A, B, C, D designate each of the four crews of shift workers.

A SAMPLE FIXED SHIFT SCHEDULE

Days of the week

Hours working	M	T	W	T	F	S	S	M	T	W	T	F	S	S	M	T	W	T	F	S	S
7.00 a.m. – 3.00 p.m.	A*	A	A	A	A	A	D	A	A	A	A	A	D	A	A	A	A	A	D	A	A
3.00 p.m. – 11.00 p.m.	B	D	B	B	B	B	B	B	B	D	B	B	B	B	B	B	B	D	B	B	B
11.00 p.m. – 7.00 a.m.	C	C	C	C	D	C	C	C	C	C	C	C	C	D	D	C	C	C	C	C	C

* The letters A, B, C designate each of the three fixed shift crews. The letter D designates the *rotating* break shift crew.

the clearly neurotic individual (neuroticism is normally used as a description of psychological health) and others who may be unsuited for medical reasons. They should not be selected for this type of work. The unsuitability may be due to permanent or temporary social reasons, such as family problems, adult education programmes, transportation difficulty or other community responsibilities which preclude shift work. It should be appreciated that there are many different schedules for shift work ranging from the permanent day or night shift through divided day and rotating two- and three-cycle night shifts. It is with the rotating cycle shift and its constant recurring irregularity of living that complaints arise; yet others find satisfaction in this way of life, for continuous three-cycle shift workers have been found to have consistently and significantly lower sickness rates than day workers in similar occupations, both in the number of episodes of sickness and in the average annual duration of absence per man. Dr. Peter Taylor, who has made many studies into the problems of shift work, suggests ". . . that the main reasons for the difference . . . lie in the degree of personal involvement in the work and in the social structure of the working group". In effect this means a greater degree of job satisfaction in these self-selected individuals, who may claim that they can plan their social activities ahead, such as working outdoors in the garden in daylight in all seasons; they can take the family out in off-peak periods and find there is less traffic congestion when going to work. It is beyond my brief to go further into the detailed design of shift schedules but I have included a table of the currently used systems. Explanation of the differential use of these can be found in standard references.

Thus you will see that it is no easy task to pronounce on the effects of shift work: man is an individual and will respond as an individual to stress; to some the stress of shift work is a stimulus and challenge, to others a dreaded chore. The answer must eventually lie somewhere between the selection, preferably by the worker himself, and the education of people to see the need for this method of fully utilising industrial plant and other kind of expensive or necessary equipment so as to obtain the maximum benefit for the community at large.

7 The Human Frame: Design for Working

The human bony and cartilaginous skeleton together with the muscles which, as well as enveloping it, have also helped to shape it, continues in a state of evolution. It still retains vestiges in the coccyx bone, of the tail of the nut-gathering apes which use both tail and arms to swing above ground. The larger brain capacity of the higher apes and earliest humans dictated that the lower limb should take precedence as means of locomotion and that, not satisfied with waddling and shuffling as do the higher apes, man also wanted to run and jump, requiring increased leg length. The extended leg length of certain desert and savannah mammals and marsupials is a parallel example on another phylogenetic plane. The upright posture modified the function of the bony spine which became lengthened but, unless firmly supported by muscles, more unstable. Only when clothed in strong muscles and ligaments can this vital organ, the human spine, perform the co-ordinated crane-like actions required of it, pivoting from the potentially unstable hip joints. The spine and thighs together, when in perfect position and mechanically integrated, act as crane and hoist allowing man to lift more than his own weight again and again without damage or discomfort. The human frame is in constant dynamic equilibrium, growth and decay balancing each other delicately provided the tasks it is asked to perform are carried out correctly, in sequence and within its mechanical capacity: it is in fact the stress stimulus of effort itself which promotes growth. Throughout life the nature and degree of these tasks will differ, or should do so, allowing time for learning and readjustment, to avoid too rapid a "normal" process of degeneration, not to speak of frank damage from acute overload.

49

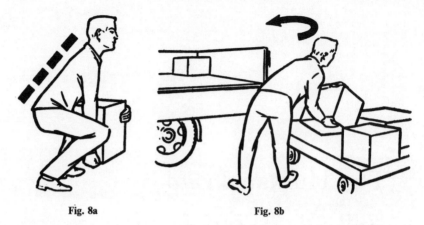

Fig. 8a   Fig. 8b

Fig. 8 a, b *How loads should be lifted and carried.* When lifting the operator must lower his body by bending his knees at right angles, without bending his back, and keep the object as near to him as possible (fig. 8a). The operator must have sufficient space to have freedom of movement and place his feet on solid and stable parts. If the object to be lifted is box-shaped it must be grasped by two diagonally opposed top ends and the corner nearest to his body placed between his legs. When lifting and placing down the load, the object should not be at his side to prevent straining the vertebral column (fig. 8b).

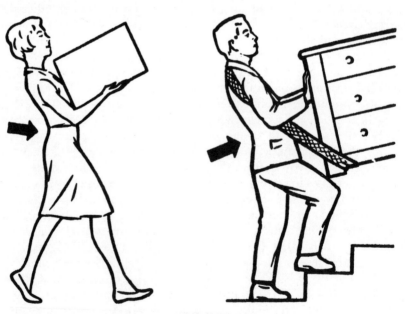

Fig. 9

Fig. 9 He should not bend his body when carrying.

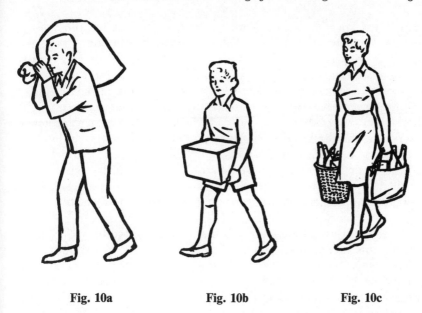

Fig. 10a   Fig. 10b   Fig. 10c

Fig. 10 a, b, c The centre of gravity of the load should be as near as possible to the vertical line of the carrier.

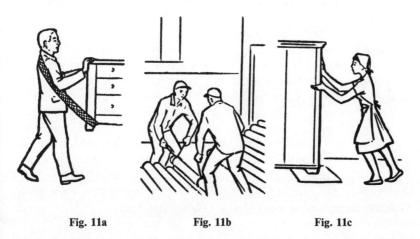

Fig. 11a   Fig. 11b   Fig. 11c

Fig. 11 a, b, c For transporting heavy loads, make use of auxiliary means to facilitate the work. Figures 8–11, from '*Maximum Permissible Weights to be carried by one worker.*' *I.L.O Geneva, 1964.*

I have used this example of the spine to illustrate the problems which can arise from mechanically imperfect use of any part of the human frame either at one moment in time or repeated over months and years but to a lesser degree. Many were the deformities which once were the accepted lot of manual workers until recently.

The "beat knee" of the coal-miner, the deformed finger joints of the window-cleaner, the calloused and dislocated joint on top of the shoulder in draymen and piano-movers – the list is very long; many of these were neither serious nor particularly painful and interfered little with gainful employment. But some conditions cruelly crippled youngsters before they were full-grown men and women – the horrors of child labour have already been alluded to in Chapter 4.

Today, thankfully, there is almost universal awareness of the need to temper performance with economy of effort and avoidance of strain: to do this requires a modicum of training in the action to be carried out, seasoned where possible with care and forethought in the design of appliances and tools needed to assist or perform the major part of the work.

With the development of automatic and semi-automatic equipment, the mechanical function of the human frame has been increasingly replaced by machines programmed to carry out complicated actions and sequences, but nonetheless requiring measures to be taken from time to time to keep them properly working whether by direct observation of the moving parts or by information fed back on dials, gauges and other kinds of recording instruments. Thus the human senses began to play an increasingly important part to the exclusion of the kinetic body movement element: this itself had built-in dangers, for the lack of physical stimulus led to sluggishness in reaction time, loss of discrimination and failure of normal replacement growth. It was therefore necessary to consider the nature and design of signals which would be continulusly acceptable and not lead to boredom and loss of attention. Not only this, but improperly designed equipment could actually create a situation where the senses, particularly the visual and auditory, were lulled into insensibility. This is illustrated vividly by the phenomenon of "flicker-fusion" when certain people, on observing the revolutions of a wheel, propeller or other rapidly circulating object, may become confused, nauseated or sleepy and even go on to have an epileptic convulsion. This reaction is probably due to the inadvertent synchronisation of the "flicker" rate with the rhythm of the normal brain waves – some people with overt or latent epileptic tendency will respond in this way. The danger is stressed of accidentally producing a lapse of awareness which could lead to disaster – indeed it has on many occasions in the past.

Like many of the recent developments resulting in improved human well-being and welfare, the understanding of the functional and economic interplay of human engineering and individual biological factors was first observed in wartime and has continued to accrue from the subsequent developments in electronics, material dynamics and human physiology studies required for government programmes, particularly atomic energy, flying, submarines, space-flight and defence against bacteriological and other forms of warfare. In this country what amounts to the successful engineering or gearing of the human frame and nervous system to the current needs is known as ergonomics and has become a fully emancipated subject in its own right, though leaning heavily on a number of disciplines to provide it with the necessary human or mechanical – in the widest sense – supporting data.

One of the current problems is that the education many of us received in youth did not prepare us for the rate of change we would experience in mid-century and beyond. We are conservative animals and the accelerating physical and psychological demands create quite severe strain – this can show itself in a number of different ways: our present climate of industrial strife and sickness absenteeism may well represent a major contribution. Perhaps more analagous are the somatic manifestations of the "dis-ease" which many people today find in their occupational environment. The significant problem of low back strain in industry is no doubt directly connected with the element of mismanagement of tasks involving the improperly co-ordinated use of back, pelvic and thigh muscles; but what is not so obvious is why some people succumb to their symptoms while others, apparently exposed to similar stresses, do not. Ergonomics cannot explain this, but it may help to reduce the problem if people set about doing things the correct way. The proper application of ergonomics presupposes a systems-analysis approach in effective functioning and in the anticipation of strains and accidents which might occur.

The human frame has much variety, but until the need arose to fit it to a restricted space, such as in aircraft, tanks, submarines and space-craft, little interest was taken in these varieties apart from some basic anthropometric studies, what came to be called somatotypes, in relation to physical and psychiatric disease characteristics. Yet there must be a wealth of material in the old army cavalry records, of fitting men to horses and horses to men; the selection of who were to be lancers and who dragoons. From the former observations, how-every, developed an awareness, not only of the subtle physical differences between people but some ideas as to how these variations, whether in their tendency to develop one form of disease more than another or in their psychological associations, restricted or enhanced a person's ability to succeed in a task and ultimately in life itself.

All of us must be familiar with the discomfort of a poorly designed chair or car seat – the effect of such discomfort, experienced day after day, on efficiency can be imagined if extrapolated to a repetitive job.

E

This question of design is as important in relation to working clothes and environment as it is to machine design: yet the protective equipment which is provided to reduce the hazard of accident and injury is itself often poorly designed and coarse and uncomfortable to wear, reducing its effectiveness and interfering with dexterity so that the worker may refuse to wear it.

While accepting the importance of these static human frame measurements, of equal value are the space, reach, grip and visual analogues; but it must be emphasised that in designing machines and work space the actual population using them should be considered. This is a difficult task today with changing labour forces and immigration. Geographical differences in man sizes are as notorious within a single country as internationally; add to this language and dialect problems and the task becomes virtually impossible for the average employer who does not possess the physical and economic facilities to effect a proper integration, though he might well realise the need. Many employers have not been aware of these difficulties: as recently as 1969 in a large government department, to wit the G.P.O., selection of candidates for mail driving and postal delivery was not influenced by their physique.

One must emphasise that the most effective way to achieve a successful movement or operation is through the application of ergonomic principles; to remind us of the original Greek meaning, this is the customs, habits and laws of work. From such apparently simple data as the leg length required to reach the rudder bar of a high-speed combat aircraft, the whole concept of the design and position of levers and instruments in relation to body measurement and conformation, psychological status and environment conditions, has been developed. Thus the applied physiologist, psychologist and anthropoligist have emerged as significant factors in both military and civilian technical development.

Elsewhere we have described the circadian rhythms of the human body (Chapter 6): it is also the economic control and output of human energy which require the application of rhythmic principles to muscle and nerve so as to achieve a balanced physiological and psychological harmony: practitioners of yoga have long known this. Biological dysrhythmia of the internal body environment is unsettling and exhausting whether of brain, heart or bowel: physiological rhythm is usually not noticeable and the individual is seldom continuously aware of it. An analogy from the working environment can be recognised in the almost beautiful rhythmic movements a master bricklayer or a plasterer makes, or more rarely today, the labourer with a scythe; all a joy to watch and remarkably untiring. While speed of work is important it must be carefully regulated to

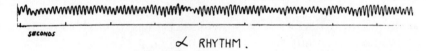

∝ RHYTHM.

Fig. 12 Electro-encephalograph tracing, showing normal alpha rhythm of the Brain (Many waves per second). (*Courtesy of Dr. C. C. Evans.*)

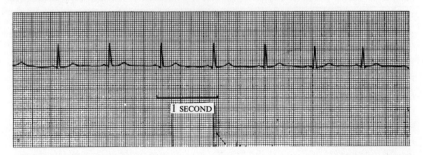

Fig. 13 An Electrocardiograph tracing showing the normal rhythm of the heart. (About one wave per second.)

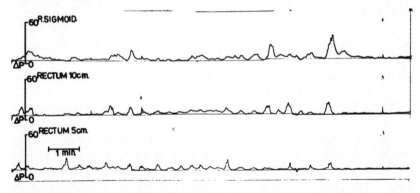

Fig. 14 Bowel rhythm: rhythmic contractions of the lower portions of the human large intestine. (About 3 waves per minute.) (*Courtesy of Dr. Sheila Waller.*)

avoid errors and accidents: the order in which movements are made will reduce fatigue and complement the optimum speed. Man is not an automaton and his movements are governed by his perception of the information reaching him, its recognition, interpretation and final translation into purposive co-ordinated movements, many of them in this technological age being fine movements of hand and eye requiring rigid concentration.

The integrative nervous system, as defined by Charles Sherrington (1857–1952) determines the speed and rhythm of work, but itself is very sensitive to feed-back information so that it can rapidly improve or lose its function. An example of this may be the ill-understood but nevertheless apparently real effect of the Chinese practice of acupuncture analgesia which, in some as yet unexplainable manner, interrupts the established afferent sensory pathways to achieve intense and remote stimulation of nerve centres while dampening the central perception of pain. In the context of what we are discussing, it would be theoretically possible to work somebody to death without his feeling any adverse effects!

The clarity of communication, whether by ear, eye or feel, is of tremendous importance: the latter sense, still much relied upon, has necessitated an intricate cybernetic technology to be developed to provide the appropriate stimulation in a variety of mechanical processes. A recent illustration of the need for application of ergonomics to daily living has been the tragedies on the motorways during fog – there is some factor or factors which have been overlooked in the training of drivers, the design of motor cars and the environmental engineering of the roadways. "For example, large amounts of data are rapidly conveyed through the medium of vision, but only of course if the subject happens to be looking in the right direction at the time that the information appears. Conveyance of information by sound is usually slower but has the advantage that the subject's attention can be attracted, whichever way he is looking. A well-designed system might therefore make use of sound signals to direct attention to particular parts of a display, in which detailed information could rapidly be given. A further important matter with regard to indicators is that data which have to be accumulated over a period of time may often be lost. This is especially so when data have to be carried in "short-term" memory while some other activity took place. It seems desirable, therefore, that whatever information has to be conveyed should, other things being equal, be conveyed at once." While these words were written some years before the emergence of motorways in this country, their relevance to our modern nose-to-tail high-speed travel on motorways is surely unmistakeable.

Perhaps one of the most important aspects of work safety and economy is standardisation, whether of indicators, wiring, design of machines, safety mechanisms, lubrication points or a host of other factors which make for ease and comfort of operation. But within this standardisation there must be room for the adaptation of equipment to an acceptable percentage of the worker population.

While we have rightly placed the emphasis on "fitting the job to the man", the antithesis is not to be overlooked even in these enlightened days. Training has been touched upon in an earlier section, but the physiological application of mechanics to human muscular activity and effort is of vital importance, particularly in the field of weight-lifting, carrying, climbing, pushing and handling awkward and heavy goods. There are, unfortunately, wide gaps in the training of all sections of our population and thus it is not surprising that back and skeletal troubles comprise a major proportion of industrial morbidity statistics; back pain was recently found to be ". . . responsible for some 60 per cent of sickness absence due to rheumatism . . . rheumatic complaints result in some 30 million lost work days every year in Britain and a loss of £150 million in wages alone". It has been said that the advent of the mini-skirt would be marked for posterity by the disappearance of low back pain in women – their method of bending to pick up objects from the ground suddenly reveals (amongst other things) a real appreciation of physiological principles!

What the employer needs are some clear, simple guides by which he can satisfy a reasonable variety of individuals' needs and, most important, be seen to be concerned and active about the working comfort of his employees.

1. Displays of information should be clear, unambigous and reduced to the simplest data required for an operation.
2. There should be sufficient but not too much light: the colours of controls and background should be carefully thought out and acceptable. The colour schemes of the total environment are well worth careful assessment and design.
3. Hand and foot controls should be as consistent as possible on as many machines as possible: they should be within the range of the majority of his current worker population and he should take care to select out those workers who are too large or too small. The power required for manipulation of the controls should similarly be adjusted for his workers.
4. Working clothes should be properly designed, fitted, clean and in good repair.
5. Protective equipment must be provided and worn when required and should be well designed, light, aesthetically acceptable in the case of women particularly, and not interfere with the proper carrying out of the job, sometimes over prolonged periods.
6. Adverse environmental conditions such as temperature, humidity, noise, vibration, ozone production, oil mists; proximity of other workers or interfering power cables and other structures should be avoided.
7. Advice is available from a number of sources.*

* See Appendix.

APPENDIX

Sources of information concerning ergonomics.

The Factory Inspectorate.

The Industrial Society,
48 Bryanston Square, London, W.1.
Tel.: 262–2401

The Royal Society for the Prevention of Accidents,
6 Buckingham Place, London, S.W.1.
Tel.: 828–7444

The Ergonomics Information Analysis Centre,
Dept. of Engineering Production,
University of Birmingham

The Ergonomics Research Society,
R. G. Sell, Esq., Hon. General Secretary,
c/o Phillips Industries,
Central Personnel Department,
Berkshire House, High Holborn,
London, W.C.1, V 7 AQ

8 The Natural History of Accidents

The human's proclivity for accidents is almost unique, perhaps his only near rival being the ape and then only when away from its natural haunts. Previous chapters have dealt successively with the behaviour and progress of people at their work and the influence of the many factors which bear on the happiness, progress and satisfaction in producing something or providing a service. The pathway through a working life will often be treacherous and sometimes dangerous as a result of the fallibilities of masters and men, changing economic climates in the national and international sphere and not least the paces, patterns and materials of work to which people may be slow to adapt and to which they may exhibit individual sensitivity.

It is fair to say that the clearest marker of tolerance to a given situation, whether at work or at home, is the ability with which a person can handle either novel tools or experience without injuring themselves or others. Despite all the success of medical science and its more recent analogue – social science – men, women and children continue to suffer more than any other ill from injuries sustained in the home, at play and at work.

This is true of people in all climates and at all times of their life: we have plenty of documentary evidence of the sad state of affairs over the last 7,000 years, and the process continues in those of our brothers still experiencing the most primitive ways of life in Australia, New Guinea, Africa and South America. We have ourselves witnessed the tragedies of astronautics, man's most recent venture, and have come to accept the calculated risk when weighed against the benefits of rapid intercontinental traffic and telecommunications. A reciprocal relationship existed until recently between the intricacy of an act and the actuality of an accident: it used to depend on the skill acquired, through training, of those operating complex equipment. There is now a danger, and indeed some indication that while complexity of equipment continues to increase, the skill and knowledge for its safe handling may not meet the demand: we have seen this happen recently in the complicated task of air traffic handling.

In this country a continual watch and record is kept of work accidents and these are analysed at regular intervals by government departments, industrial safety organisations, and individual firms' safety committees where they exist. Our laws are now being reviewed to increase the responsibility of both employer and employee towards the control of work accidents; these must also include the control of environment and the selection and training of workers. The design of machinery and operations with safety considerations incorporated remains perhaps the most important need and their current inadequacies continue to exploit the element of human failure. Nevertheless the incorporation of systems to offset the frailties of human behaviour, function and physique has benefited from developments in other spheres; increasingly we are seeing pre-set operations being introduced at the level of the shop floor. But for many years to come the too gradual re-tooling of our engineering industry will continue to provoke the worker into acts of stupidity which attempts to "design out" in the past have never fully succeeded in preventing.

There are legal requirements for the incorporation of special guards on machinery; these may be "fixed" to prevent any interference with the mechanism or "automatic" in the sense that the machine cannot operate unless all human contact has been withdrawn from the working mechanism. Various forms of "fail-safe" systems exist such as the "interlock" which prevents any operation until the mechanism is in correct starting position – these are increasingly used in a variety of machines from motor cars with car-seat belts to micro-wave ovens, both being examples of the non-industrial use of safety equipment. "Trip" guards are needed where frequent interference is required as in small roller-mill and guillotine operations.

The psychological aspects of handling dangerous machinery are brought home to us in considering the appalling havoc wrought by fog on the motor-ways in this country – until now the awareness of "normal" or more correctly "usually expected" signals enables a person to react either deliberately or involuntarily which will reflect training and experience. It has been wisely said that "reliance should not be placed on copious instructions for the correct use of equipment. The answer is to design machines and equipment that cannot have liberties taken with them." Extrapolate this to the design of motor cars and you see the size of the problem in the total context of human injury through accidents.

The nature and incidence (frequency of new episodes) of accidents at work will depend upon many factors, not least the attitude and peace of mind of the worker at work. The point was put topically when the tabloid of the British Safety Council, *Safety and Rescue*, in its July 1972 number reported the opinion of the safety officer from a Durham coal-mine that "A morning kiss and a cuddle from his wife can ensure that a miner returns home safely at the end of his shift". His view is shared by the miners at his colliery. Having "something on the mind" is within the experience of all of us and its effect upon concentration can be both momentary or prolonged over a period during which the whole behaviour may become altered, resulting in a series of episodes: this factor is touched upon later, but now we are concerned with the physical and environmental influences which result in a very wide scatter of both the frequency of accidents and their nature. Again, personal experience must colour our appreciation of and action to forestall accident. Some are fortunate to have none, others to be either susceptible themselves or observe it in others. The experience gained in heavy engineering, mining and elsewhere cannot fail to impress responsible people. Even the "Acts of God" such as electrocution by lightning should bring home to people the need to take all reasonable precautions to avoid injury. To this end the training of safety officers, of first-aid workers, the establishment of rescue teams and disaster plans are aimed. But none of these can replace the important aspect of the individual well trained in his job. Facilities now exist throughout the whole country for all of these, but remain on a voluntary basis as far as the individual worker or employer is concerned, although a statutory requirement under the Factories Acts is the establishment of a fully trained first-aid worker in premises employing more than fifty people and the appointment of a safety supervisor in a similar situation under the Building Regulations.

Perhaps I cannot emphasise the differing patterns of accidents better than to review their geographical distribution and incidence in this country. Earlier, in the introduction to these chapters we have seen how the industry in Britain moved away from its original home in south-east England following the discovery of coal and steam: the accompanying maps and legends show that along with this movement work accidents have become much more frequent north of a line draw from the Severn to the Wash. It is the metal, shipbuilding and marine industries which predominate: these are geographically sited in South Wales, South Yorkshire and the north-east of England. On the national scale of work accidents, the stati-

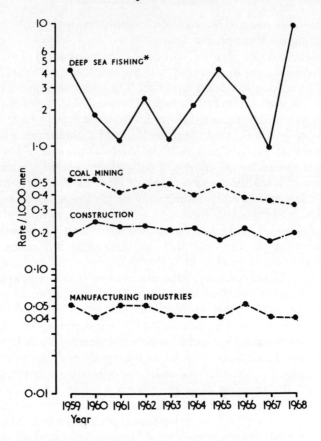

* These rates are for accidents at sea only; it is estimated that the inclusion of deaths ashore would increase these yearly rates by about 0·2 per 1000. Hazards of Deep-Sea fishing. (*R. S. F. Schilling Brit. Jour. Indust. Med. 28.27.35. 1971.*)

Fig. 15 Fatal accident rates per 1000 men at risk. (Sources—Registrar General Shipping and Seamen; Medical Statistics Branch National Coal Board; H.M. Factory Inspectorate.)

stically most dangerous occupations as defined by fatality figures are deep-sea fishing, agriculture and coal-mining. It was the occasion of an investigation into skin conditions among North Sea fishermen which brought the serious problem of accidents at sea to the attention of workers in occupational health: the figures had apparently been disregarded and indeed poorly documented in the annual reports of the Department of Agriculture and Fisheries: only a short while previously had the very serious toll of accidents among agricultural workers come to light.

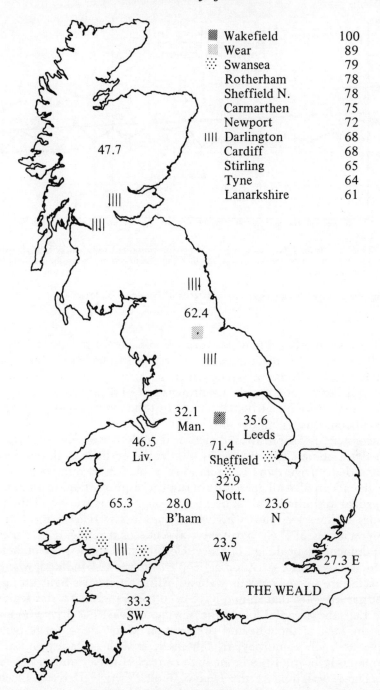

Wakefield 100
Wear 89
Swansea 79
Rotherham 78
Sheffield N. 78
Carmarthen 75
Newport 72
Darlington 68
Cardiff 68
Stirling 65
Tyne 64
Lanarkshire 61

47.7

62.4

32.1
Man.

35.6
Leeds

46.5
Liv.

71.4
Sheffield

32.9
Nott.

65.3

28.0
B'ham

23.6
N

23.5
W

27.3 E

THE WEALD

33.3
SW

Fig. 16 Relative frequency of reported accidents in factory processes—a geographical sample. (Taken from Annual Rep. Chief Inspect. Factories 1968 HMSO)

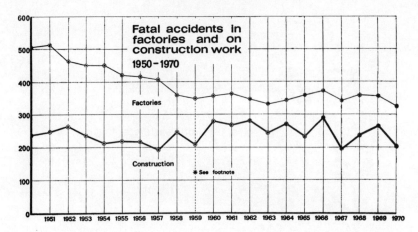

Fatal accidents in factories and on construction work 1950–1970

Factories

Construction

* See footnote

* The figures from 1960 onwards include fatalities reported from works brought within the scope of the Factories Act by the Engineering Construction (Extension of Definition) Regulations 1960 and 1968.

Fig. 17 (*Annual Report 1971 Chief Inspector of Factories, HMSO.*)

Yet when all accidents at work are considered together, they are still exceeded by the tragedies occurring during leisure hours and in the home itself, many of which go unrecorded: each year in Britain some 1,200 people are drowned at play and sport and 7,000 die from accidents at home. Taken in terms of a threat to people's livelihood, this is considerable and has been steadily increased by the introduction of sophisticated electrical and other equipment into the modern home. The frequency of deaths of little children inside discarded refrigerators is, unhappily, a marker of affluence. Home accidents involve all ages and consume a disproportionate amount of medical and nursing time because of their concentration at the two poles of life. The ease with which they occur reflects the lack of appreciation of their possibility, absence of training in the use of equipment, poor design of space, clothing and the variety of factors which distract the attention of people from the task in hand, whether it is failure to concentrate when adjusting an electric light fitting or the greater care that should have been taken in fixing a stair-carpet. Perhaps the dreadful toll on the new motor-ways has driven home to us the lack of thought and preparation which the average person gives to such a journey, fraught as it is with so many situations apparently beyond the immediate control of driver and passengers.

The redesigning of the Heavy Goods Vehicle Driver's Licence requirements, particularly the medical examination, has gone some of the way to screen out men who might be a danger to themselves and others, but as yet its influence has been little felt since the innovation in February 1970. Nevertheless, the health of drivers of these increasingly complicated vehicles imposes a major responsibility on those on whom the decision falls when the time comes for appraisal. The nature of the work, the absence of sufficient bodily exercise to restrict the onset of obesity, a natural sequence of the way of life of many truck drivers, their diets restricted to greasy, carbohydrate-loaded meals, the consumption of large quantities of beer, all of these combine to decrease efficiency, watchfulness and quick reaction to emergency situations. In itself the problems of heavy duty transport drivers is a major issue and, beyond bringing it to general attention, must remain beyond our present consideration.

So far we can say that sufficient motivation, education, maturity, equipment and alertness are the basic requirements of the well-equipped worker today. Education for future work should commence at a receptive age, and this could well mean that school curricula should be designed to introduce safe practices in home and the working environment, in a general sense. The new Industrial Training Boards have assumed a considerable significance in this field although the results of their efforts may not be reflected for some years. The potential worker then is the natural point to which preventive methods should be aimed, provided the need and cost of them can be accepted. This presupposes a receptive attitude which must inevitably depend on the attitudes in young people's homes, their primary and secondary education, their vocational direction and training and their responsibility to society: policies of perfection which are difficult to introduce and maintain in a rapidly changing world of fashion and culture. Herein may lie the answer: there is enormous scope to harness the power and influence of current modes and mores to induce a desire to avoid illness and injury resulting from poor practice and bad environment.

Much has been written and spoken of the psychological causes of accidents: in the final event, it is human attitude and failure which influences whether a process can be complicated in this way. The recent, though not yet universal, introduction of the reporting of all accidents irrespective of whether they have caused injury or not, the so-called "damage-control", has enabled those responsible for overall prevention to identify the areas where workers attention and training should be focused. (While injuries to work people cost this country over £700 million a year, damage to plant, property, tools, equipment and materials costs seventeen times this figure.) By these means potentially dangerous situations which have not yet caused injury to workers, but which could do so if work people were more closely involved, can be studied and measures taken to reduce the chances of their recurrence in which a man or woman might this time be injured.

As in other fields involving the observation and actions of numbers of people, it is the "inevitable 10 per cent" who seem to be the ones more likely to have accidents resulting in injury. This is brought out by the study of accident records both within plants themselves and through the payment of insurance claims: it has been clearly shown that defects in the behavioural attitudes of people having repreated accidents can be tied to their personality, in its turn dependent or influenced by factors not necessarily consistently involving the work situation directly, but bearing some relation to inter-personal relationships at the level of management and in the social and domestic milieu away from work.

While accidents are legally notifiable if disability from them lasts more than three days, the resultant statistics do not measure safety performance, which is too sensitive to other factors. The only stable factor is the fatal accident. Experience has taught us in medicine that the multifactorial approach to diagnosis of cause and effect of mental and physical illness pays the best dividends and the *modus operandi* should be the same when investigating the cause of both a single accident or the problem of repeated accidents in the same individual. Once again we return to the point where education, selection and training are the linchpins which are required to hold together all the other influences which, if allowed to express themselves unevenly, can result in acts of ignorance, stupidity, carelessness and wilfulness.

Thus the problem of accidents is seen to be influenced from three main directions – the individual, the local environment and the picture throughout the whole country. Undoubtedly the continuous campaigns against industrial accidents have succeeded in improving the standard of reporting which is reflected to an extent in the figures over the years, which do not show as satisfactory a fall as could be hoped for. The situation is still disappointing as those who have reviewed the problem in depth have recently remarked: "It is not apparent that there has been any significant reduction in the size of the problem as a whole although there have been variations in the incidence of particular hazards as a result of specialised attack."

The Chief Inspector of Factories has lately given a slightly more optimistic picture: he points out that the application of legal restraints, coupled with the efforts by the industries themselves in training and education, have brought considerable improvement over a period of nearly forty years. This is illustrated by the earlier figures for "Factory Processes" before the 1937 Factories Act, taken against the comparable figures today. The average incidence rate per 100,000 employed in the period 1929–38 was 11·6: by 1970 these had fallen to 4·5. However, we cannot be complacent because the character of accidents is changing with the increasing use of mechanical aids as instanced by transportation accidents in the factories, which are now the largest single cause of fatal accidents. Bear in mind that this does not measure the immediate and long-term disablement problems for employees or employers of those involved in a non-fatal accident.

The battle then has been joined by industry itself through the training and authority given to safety officers, the Industrial Training Boards and the safety organisations, in particular the Royal Society for the Prevention of Accidents and the British Safety Council. Legislation may shortly be further extended to put the responsibility in the hands of both workers and management. Continuous contact is maintained with international bodies similarly concerned; the scope for accidents and ill-effects of occupation increases along with the introduction of highly sophisticated techniques. However, prevision has at last entered the thinking of those responsible for their design and introduction: the last redoubt, the users' ignorance and disregard, is now being tackled with some hope of success.

It is not easy to summarise the problem and any summary by definition cannot be comprehensive.

1. *The law* requires all accidents causing absence from work of three days or longer to be reported. It also provides, through a system of inspectors, advice and if necessary, prosecution and a system of fines; persuasion not prosecution is the guiding principle however.

2. *The worker:* primary and secondary education of the child and youth should incorporate safety principles.

Training for work: Industrial training boards.
Apprenticeships.
Induction periods.
Selection

Health Alertness Motivation Accident history.
Safety education: posters, pamphlets, personal responsibility, safety committees, safety officers, exhibitions, films, clothing, hair, finger nails, etc.

3. *The job:* Main fields of work: home, school, offices, shops, laboratories, hospitals, transport, light and heavy industry, mines, fisheries, agriculture.

Design of machine and methods of operation.
Design of tackle and implements.
Guards.
Storage, stacking and scaffolding.
Production speed.

4. *The environment:* Indoors, outdoors.

Weather   Temperature   Ventilation   Lighting

Fatigue ————— | ————— Good vision

Wet slippery hands

Housekeeping: Electric cables.
Water spillage.
Slippery floor.
Plant and machinery maintenance.
Jagged metal edges.
Obstruction of through-ways.
Flying foreign bodies (grinding,
chiselling, welding, cooling metal).
Holes in the floor.
Dust

Respiratory discomfort   skin irritation   explosion

Design of protective equipment and its
enforcement.
Escape of gases.

9 The Nature of Occupational Health Disorders

It is of more than passing interest that many of today's disorders once lay well within the limits of normal health; indeed, they continue to do so for a large proportion of the world's population. We can cite hookworm infestation, menopausal problems, protein deficiency, alcoholism, multiple pregnancies, senility and dental caries as a few examples of what is still too long a list. But one by one, as they have become recognised as conditions that should be treated and prevented, they are no longer acceptable in our society. In the same manner changes have occurred in other walks of life; head and body lice are not *persona grata* in high society, nor is subsistence farming tolerated in a sophisticated community. They are now recognised as markers of underdevelopment because they have failed to meet the ideals and rising expectations of society.

Disorder emphasises a potentially reversible disturbance of the physiological or psychological balance of the organism or cell, in distinction to the actual structural pathology which predicates disease. To avoid semantic confusion we can say that much of the recognised disease of today was yesterday's disorder, thanks to refined methods of revealing structural, biochemical and now molecular and chromosomal changes. Almost daily, with the development of new biological techniques, the pictures of many disorders of the past are being clarified into systematic pathology: consumption becomes pulmonary tuberculosis; the ague becomes malaria, rickets becomes vitamin D deficiency, a significant proportion of patients with senile dementia are recognised as myxoedema (thyroid deficiency) and so on, as we advance.

F

Yet many of the symptoms which cause people at work to complain or absent themselves don't seem to have any clinically recognisable basis, either of cause or effect. This is the enigma which bedevils our understanding and handling of these problems, particularly when the means of objective assessment, either biologically in the body and its products or in the environment at work, are not practicable. This may be because of expense, technical deficiency or reluctance to use the facilities which do exist.

If environmental pollution, whether ideological or by noise, gasses, dusts, fumes and aerosols are allowed to act upon a person he will react depending upon his individual susceptibility. Only in recent years have we begun to understand why the reactions of different people to pleasurable or noxious stimuli from physical, chemical and biological agents vary over such a wide range and themselves may be dependent upon changing influences in the same individual. Here are some well-known examples to illustrate this: differing thresholds for pain, inborn variations in taste, reaction to toxic effects of lead, mercury, some solvents and ethyl alcohol; exposure to certain chemicals causing haemolysis (rupture of red blood cells) and muscle paralysis. These emphasise that it is at the level of cell metabolism and energy transfer catalysed by enzymes where much of the individual differences lie. These disorders are only the tip of the iceberg, the main body of which will come into view as new and more accurate methods of analysis are developed. The alternative and more attractive possibility, that the iceberg will dissolve and disappear, is most unlikely because of the constant introduction of new, potentially dangerous materials reinforcing it, as it were, from below: the mutation rate of human genes cannot keep pace with the changing environment. Dr. Charles Fletcher points the real issue: "In studying a person's health, we are inclined to compare it with the so-called normal. The trouble is that one cannot speak of normal other than by reference to a single biological constant. The concept of a normal individual in medicine, is linked to the fact that clinical and laboratory examinations made at a point in time, do not indicate the presence of a morbid entity, and anatomical biochemical and psychological measurements are found to be within the limits accepted as normal. Thus the error in pronouncing an individual normal consists of the minute number of investigated parameters as compared with their real number. Moreover these parameters are established in their static aspect, a disadvantage which can be proved by a tolerance test studying the dynamic equilibrium of a given process."

The image of occupational disorders is so broad that its borders merge imperceptibly into general medical conditions not usually considered to bear a relation to the daily working environment. Let me give one or two examples:

1. *Obesity.* A 29-year-old manager of a packaging firm who weighed 161 kg. (308 lb.). His weight had increased 50 kg. (128 lb.) over a period of five years while he was employed, after leaving school at the age of 17, on the manufacturing floor of a chocolate factory: he tested the products freely. Obesity is an occupational hazard of confectioners, publicans and pastry cooks.

2. *Myocardial Infarction* (Coronary thrombosis.) Recent epidemiological studies have shown the relation between myocardial infarction and men working in the viscose rayon industry. Those exposed over a long period to low concentrations of carbon disulphide (CS_2) have shown a significant increase in frequency above the expected rate for this disease.

3. *Arthritis and Bone Necrosis.* (Local death of bone tissue.) These may arise some time after episodes of decompression sickness in tunnellers and others exposed to high (compressed) air pressures, usually above 35 lb./sq. inch. Notification of episodes of decompression sickness has not been effective in the past and a patient may not consider his occupational history significant.

4. *Cataract.* Lens opacities occur after prolonged exposure to infrared radiation in furnace men, foundry workers and others handling red-hot material such as glass, and have been suspected to arise following non-ionising radiation with very high frequency radiowaves (microwaves). The degenerative and metabolic causes of cararact are not easy to separate from the occupational, especially when the exposure has been remote in time.

5. *Hydatid Disease.* (Parasitic worm cysts in the tissues.) This was once a well-recognised condition in Lebanese shoe-makers who used to prepare leather by soaking it in a mixture of water and dog's faeces! The dogs in the Middle East are heavily infested with the intestinal worm *Echinococcus granulosus*. It is well to remember that bacterial and parasitic infections in certain populations may have a close connection with occupation.

These cautionary tales illustrate the approach which should always be made to expose an occupational factor in an illness, whether it appears to be of toxic, infective, neoplastic or degenerative origin. What do you do? For how long have you done it? How do you do it? What materials do you use? Do you know of special precautions you should have taken? What were your previous occupations? Have any of your work-mates been sick with a similar complaint?

From the answers to these questions it might be wise to dwell at some length on the conditions of the patient's work, but caution is needed because careful investigation will be required before accepting any connection. Statistically the chances of finding overt occupational diseases are slight in these enlightened days, although they certainly do occur as witnessed by the story of acrylamide poisoning described by Garland and Patterson from this hospital, and the more recent episode of lead absorption from the smelting plant in Avonmouth.

Until the Second World War the health of people in this country had shown wide and regional variations, stemming from the slow improvement in the control of communicable disease, the disparity of nutritional intakes and the diverse and often wretched conditions in which the people had lived during the great population expansion of the nineteenth and early twentieth centuries. The potentiating effect of bad environmental conditions on a physique already strained by malnutrition and repeated illness was only too apparent: the spectre of tuberculosis stalked the land and we now know the influence which certain dusts of occupational origin had on the activation of this formerly widespread disease, when deposited in the lung. Perhaps nothing is more striking to the returning wanderer who has been away from this country for thirty years than to see the remarkable change in the standard of physical health enjoyed by industrial workers. One cannot help but wonder how much this has contributed to the low incidence of overt industrial disease, aided by the control of environment and processes brought about by the Factories Acts. While the susceptibility of the main body of people has decreased among less-favoured individuals, genetically determined idiosyncrasies, mostly enzymic in nature, may actually have increased. Unfortunately we have little idea of the change in individual biochemical and physiological profiles resulting from the effects of age, sex, race, exercise, diet and seasonal variations, nor have we the means of knowing when these profiles first begin to be distorted by the earliest effects of an unfriendly environment. We are beholden, in the main, to subjective reactions and usually only late objective phenomena. Nevertheless, there are now some signs of a breakthrough in being able to recognise the biochemical individuality which all of us possess. With the forward march of science and the development of newer and no less dangerous materials the body has continuously to learn to adjust; we know that certain people are better at this than others and in some cases we know why. A number of these materials are well known and in common industrial use, such as parathion, benzene, carbon-tetrachloride, trichlorethylene, arsine (AsH_2), nitrogen oxides, lead, cadmium, mercury, beryllium and asbestos: others are therapeutic drugs, such as butazolidine, phenobarbitone and sulpha drugs.

Adverse working conditions may increase the rate of absorption of toxic substances, if continued for any length of time. The exposure of workers to high environmental temperatures will, because of the hyperkinetic effect of the circulatory dynamics, increase absorption of some chemicals and their rate of reaction. This in turn overloads the detoxicating mechanisms of the body and reduces excretion following a slowing of the glomerular kidney filtration rate in the presence of haemo-concentration (thick viscous blood): the larger and longer turnover of the substance has a more prolonged effect upon end-organs such as the heart, kidney, liver and brain. Chemical plant operators and agricultural workers in hot countries using dangerous pesticides are particularly at risk because of the discomfort of wearing protective clothing which they may discard. This problem also arises among workers exposed to flash fires, chemical burns and intoxicating gases. Some physical factors modify the body's response to chemical and physical therapeutic agents and are utilised in medicine in such treatments as the potentiating effect on deep X-ray therapy by hyperbaric oxygen (oxygen under increased atmospheric pressure).

The standards by which industrial environments are evaluated have secured a measure of world-wide acceptance, although there are still inexplicable and considerable differences in levels between those acceptable in Russia and her satellites and the rest of the manufacturing world. Some Russian figures are more conservative by a factor of as much as ten. Before dismissing these criteria as impossibly low one should remember that Russian physiological tradition adheres to the Pavlovian theory, while in many Western countries this has long been discarded as inappropriate or even downright misleading. These views are being reconsidered particularly in the light of the success of Russian space research and modern aversion therapy in this country and America. Conditions of climate, genetic patterns and industry itself may differ widely in Russia as compared to other areas. For instance, only two years ago Western manufacturing countries preferred to accept the U.S.A. standard for microwave exposure level as 10 microwatt/cm^2 while considering the Russian standard of 1 microwatt/cm^2 "impossibly low." Yet now domestic equipment is being produced to this "impossibly low" Russian standard following widespread demands for increased safety.

The standard safe limit of pollution in an industrial environment is known as the "threshold limit value" (T.L.V.) and applies to substances which may be either injurious or offensive if absorbed as dust, vapour, aerosol or fume. It identifies a level under which nearly all workers can be exposed day after day without known adverse effect. The qualification is made that there is a wide variation in individual susceptibility, and that a small percentage of workers may experience discomfort from some substances at concentrations at or below the threshold limit. These values are for time-weighted concentrations over an 8-hour work-day and 40-hour week: they are guides only. It is appropriate to stress that the irritative effects of a substance may "initiate, promote or accelerate impairment through interaction with other chemical or biological agents", a situation with which doctors are not unfamiliar in relation to the effects of the many powerful drugs in the modern pharmacopoeia.

We come now to the system under which accidents at work and certain "Prescribed Industrial Diseases" are handled, so that measures against their occurrence and compensation to the claimant, should they arise, may be undertaken. At the present time there are forty-eight "Prescribed Diseases", brucellosis having just been added. Further additions to the list may be made from time to time and depend upon the careful consideration that must be given to all aspects of an illness including the nature of the victim's job. Certain conditions require to be satisfied before claims for injury or disablement benefit are allowed and these are clearly set out in the relevant government leaflets. A few examples will serve to illustrate the type of exposure which qualifies for compensation should a worker become disabled, having satisfied the requirements under the National Insurance (Industrial Injuries) Acts.

1. *Lead or a compound of lead.* The use or handling of, or exposure to the fumes, dust or vapour of, lead or a compound of lead, or a substance containing lead.

7. *Benzene or a homologue.* The use or handling of, or exposure to the fumes or vapour containing, benzene or any of its homologues.

18. *Gonioma kamassii (African boxwood).* The manipulation of Gonioma kamassii or any process in or incidental to the manufacture of articles therefrom.

21 (b). *Infection by Leptospira canicola.* Work at dog kennels or the care or handling of dogs.

26. Heat cataract (thickening of the lens of the eye). Frequent or prolonged exposure to rays from molten or red-hot material.

38. *Tuberculosis.* Close and frequent contact with a source of tuberculosis infection by reason of employment (a) in the medical treatment or nursing of a person or persons suffering from tuberculosis, or in a service auxiliary to such treatment or nursing.

In a short space it is not possible to enlarge further, but the reader may wish to refer to standard texts for details of these diseases or conditions with which he is not familiar. I have confined my remarks to the general environmental circumstances giving rise to illnesses.

The span of these is remarkabley wide. Many of them are familiar ingredients of people's domestic, travel and leisure environments, medical treatment, food and cosmetics; they are experienced during some time of everyone's living day, usually in amounts far below the threshold values discussed earlier.

The difficulty arises in sifting the relevant information and, as in the case of the dermatoses and allergies, this may have to be painstaking and prolonged. While this is being done the patient will need support and every effort must be made to sustain an optimistic outlook to avoid the development of an occupational neurosis.

10 Alcoholism and Industry

It can be said that at times we are the etymological victims of our own language. This is very relevant in the context of the word "disease": what this means in ordinary conversation and medical science respectively is, due to the advances of scientific medicine, subject to different interpretation.

When discussing the problem of the chronic abuse of alcohol, in distinction to its effects, it has become customary for an informed group of medical and lay people to categorise alcoholism as a disease, in the same manner that one might now consider social props such as drugs and smoking. But this is where the definition of disease leads us astray – whilst all of these are certainly a "dis-ease" of mind and of body, in the current understanding of pathology, yet all of them eventually lead to morbid physical as well as psychological derangement. This preamble is for the benefit of those people who have either not been aware that alcoholism, among other behavioural disorders, is regarded as a disease by most doctors, and many lay-men, but also for those who positively refuse to accept that it is any more than "lack of moral fibre" and requires only "the need to pull himself together".

It is a sad fact that many people and many employers amongst them turn a blind eye to the problem: yet as much as 25 per cent of any one group of workers may have a problem of alcoholism, though indeed neither the victim, his fellow workers nor his family may be aware of it.

First of all a definition, then the steps which can and should be taken to deal with the situation at as early a stage as possible, so preserving the health of the individual, the social stability of his family and his or her ability to do a job of work.

The first scientific treatise on the effects of alcohol was in 1778,

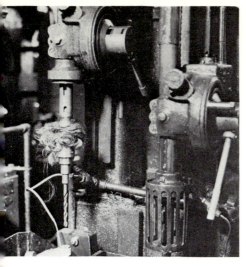

Plate 4 "The Element of Human Failure" 1.

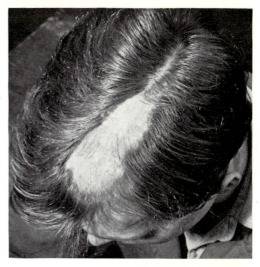

Plate 5 "The Element of Human Failure" 2.

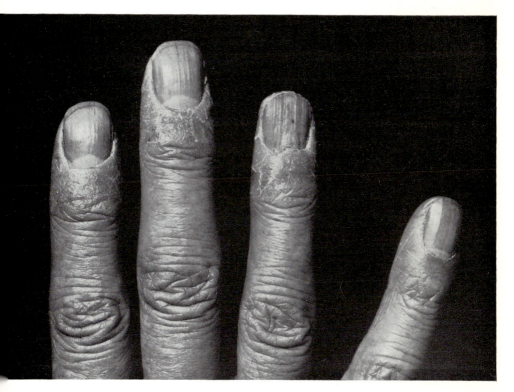

Plate 6 What do you do? How do you do it? *Rubber Dermatitis* due to wearing protective rubber fingerstalls in the book-binding industry.

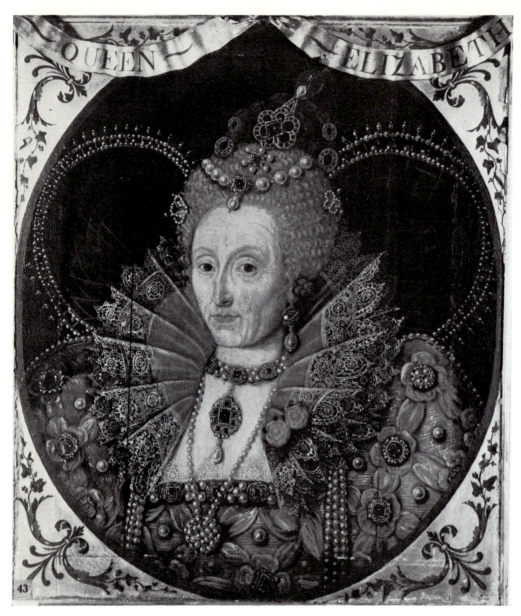

Plate 7 Queen Elizabeth 1 of England wearing her cosmetic mask of white lead oxide. Whether or not she suffered any degree of lead absorption and intoxication must remain an interesting speculation. (*Courtesy of the Courtauld Institute of Art.*)

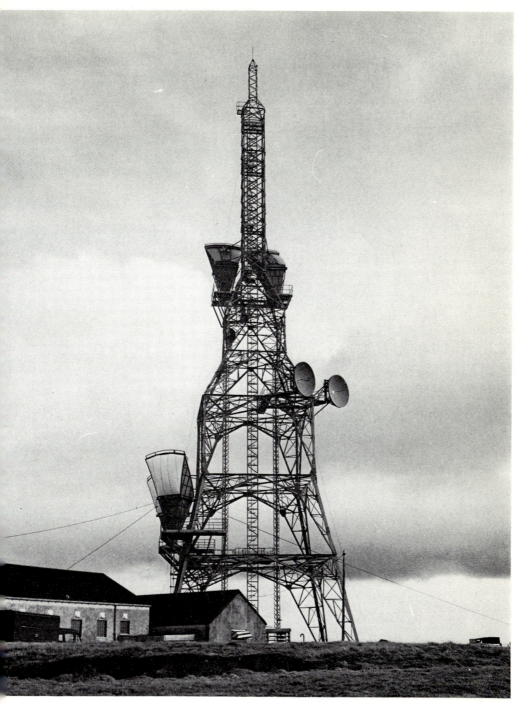

Plate 8 A micro-wave communication pylon. (*Courtesy of the Post Office.*)

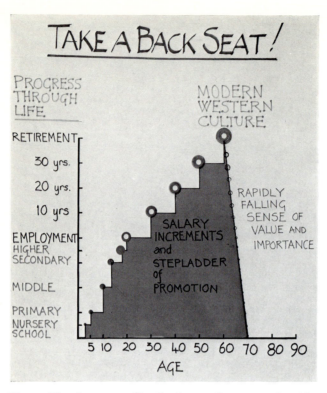

Plate 9 The abrupt cut-off at "retirement" age engendered by our present industrial culture.

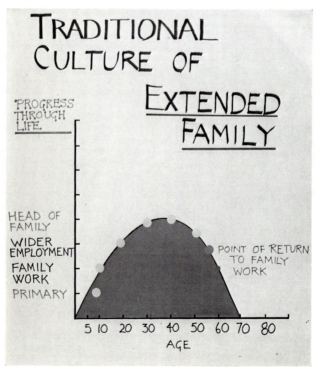

Plate 10 The life pattern hitherto in non-industrial cultures.

by Thomas Trotter, who even then defined alcoholism as a disease entity and discussed methods of treating it. It achieved much favourable attention and he was awarded a gold medal by the Humanitarian Society, but there was a long interval before alcoholism became generally recognised as a disease, only ended by studies begun in America and in particular by the group activities of "Alcoholics Anonymous".

Probably the frequency of alcoholism has actually decreased over the years if one considers the cartoons by Hogarth, Rowlandson and others and the many references to this almost general state amongst the poor and depraved following the introduction of gin at 1d. the glass, but, owing to population increase all over the world, the total number of people affected has increased. It is estimated that there are 100,000 severe alcoholics in the United Kingdom, and 500,000 ordinary alcoholics or those who sweat out their hangover without conviction for drunkness, 1 to each 100 of the population.

Everyone who is not a strict teetotaller (T-total was coined by the secretary of a New York Temperance Society, who placed T after names of those who had signed the total pledge of abstinence) has a drinking pattern influenced by several different factors: but social activities which have two main effects, a desire to be one of the boys or girls and sometimes take more than actually required, and the need for "stimulation" and relaxation of taut nerves, are probably the main ones. In effect though, this action is really a dulling of the faculty of self-criticism and the outpouring of often meaningless conversation. Again a taste for wine at meals, or a night-cap whether self-prescribed or advised by a doctor. These in moderation do no harm and perhaps good. But somewhere in that 1 per cent of the population, either from inside the body or without, arises a stimulus which will turn this moderate acceptable pattern into the pernicious and anti-social habit of heavy drinking. An old Chinese proverb has it, "First the man takes a drink; then the drink takes a drink, then the drink takes the man." Formerly, a heavy drinker was regarded as a moral degenerate, an individual who lacked "moral fibre" and was brushed off with the conclusion "once a drunk, always a drunk". This concept dies hard, but the realistic approach is to appreciate that what determines the issue is the combination of our inherited constitutional features modified by environment which are at all times susceptible to damage by outside factors. Whether that damage is sufficient to break up an established pattern of behaviour and stimulate primitive compulsions is a matter of degree, both degree of basic quality of material (constitution) and degree of exogenous stimuli.

An analogy can perhaps be drawn between the social aspects of heavy drinking today and the social ostracism of the epileptic in primitive societies. Both alcoholism and epilepsy have similarities in that they can develop in any individual at any age given a sufficient stimulus. On the one hand we can point to the problem of the juvenile alcoholic of the heavy wine-drinking countries such as France and on the other to the deliberate production of epileptic fits by electrical currents, or lack of blood supply to the brain. So we can truly say "There – but for the grace of God, go I!"

Among other causes the hereditary bases of alcoholism and epilepsy are now appreciated, and once that knowledge is gained by the individual it should, and fortunately does in many cases, act as a preventive check, teaching him to avoid those exogenous stimuli which are well known to precipitate the illness. Very similar stimuli exist for both of these conditions, fatigue, illness, over-excitement, worry and depression.

Unfortunately, unlike epilepsy it is not possible objectively to identify a potential alcoholic: in epilepsy, an electronic brain test (electroencephalogram) can identify a latent epileptic, in alcoholism this can only be done by observation after months or years of exposure to stimuli depending upon the dose and pattern of drinking; when acting together these have a greater effect than would be expected from the sum of their individual action. Once the illness progresses, and please note that I use "illness" in the very early stage of abnormal drinking, a certain recognisable character emerges, oddly enough regardless of the underlying individual character or personality: it is the cardinal features of this stage of alcoholism that those who regard it their responsibility to identify and help these people must learn to recognise.

1. A strong desire for supremacy or importance, as shown by a craving for fun and excitement, the urge to live dangerously, the inability to accept frustration, the fretting at routine or discipline – a tendency towards self-pampering ("I must have the mood I want when I want it") regardless of consequences.
2. A prevailing negative, hostile feeling – resentment, defiance, hostility are readily available on relatively slight provocation. He is constantly on the defensive about his drinking.
3. A sense of loneliness and isolation. The alcoholic generally lacks interest in anything outside himself and his problem.
4. Sexual tension and inadequacy. Many alcoholic males have never married. Of those who have, the proportion of separated and divorced is many times that in the general population.
5. The immaturity of the alcoholic is illusrtated by his rapid mood swings. From a mood in which he says to himself, "I can do nothing

I want to, or nothing is any good", he swings over to a feeling that "Everything is wonderful and I can do anything I want to".

Diagnostically the "Heavy Habit Drinker" can stop when the necessity is pointed out to him. The chronic alcohol problem drinker or addict, on the other hand, is a person who uses alcohol to such an extent that it interferes with a successful life, including physical, personality and social aspects, and he is either not able to recognise this effect or is not able to control his alcoholic consumption, although he knows its disastrous results – compare this to the stealing of a kleptomaniac and other compulsive phenomena.

The trigger required for this abnormal pattern appears so often to be alcohol itself which sets off a vicious cycle of tension and the need to relieve it.

However, it should be appreciated that there are perhaps four personality groups of individuals who may develop alcoholism, but for whom both treatment and prognosis may be different:

		What have been described as:
1. Good previous personality	–	the good
2. Underlying neurotic personality	–	the sad
3. Underlying psychotic personality	–	the mad
4. Underlying psychopathic personality	–	the bad

What sort of a problem is alcoholism in industry? This is not a question to which doctors can give a complete answer; unfortunately we tend only to see the end effects of the habit which are so disabling and pathetic; "Alcoholics and doctors don't mix", although doctors are by no means immune!

It is fair to say that most of the time most of the alcoholics in our land are at work: figures for the frequency of these people in industry vary from 1 to 26 per cent, and probably compare with those people who harbour an occult or latent diabetes but differ in that they may be identified by a screening programme. Some years ago it was possible for the medical department of a large organisation to review its problem of alcoholism; it came to know it had one unlike much of industry which does not recognise a disease which may affect a sizeable proportion of its work force. This is odd, to say the least, when the alcoholic is known to have a sickness absence record twice that of the average worker; the relevant figures are thirty days and fourteen days per annum respectively. Because the employees received total medical and health care, and because their social habits could be monitored – in this case retrospectively – in the company welfare facilities, it was possible to arrive at a rough estimate of the size of the problem and then to determine the nature of it.

The total employees numbered 2,000; of these 642 or 32 per cent were noted to be regular drinkers, 107 or 5·4 per cent to be heavy heavy drinkers, and a further small group but nonetheless very significant number 23 or 1·1 per cent were judged to be problem drinkers or alcohol addicts. It is of considerable interest that only 10 of these 23 alcoholics had in fact been identified either at work or by the medical department. Thus there were some 107 heavy drinkers and 13 addicts, a total of 120 or 6 per cent of the population who had received no medical or health advice concerning their drinking patterns. Added to this was the fact that all were skilled workers of the level of shop-foremen and above, some irreplaceable without great expense and training. A review of their work attendance records and their medical and work documents revealed the expected pattern of absenteeism and prolonged sick absences which, if the problem had been approached from that direction would have been suggestive and perhaps recognised sooner. Nevertheless, one of the biggest factors in relation to non-sick absenteeism is the element of cover-up by a man or woman's workmates. This may continue for years out of a mistaken sense of friendship and loyalty only to lead eventually to the awful physical and psychological degradation which is the final lot of the uninhibited alcoholic.

Who is the alcoholic? It could be you or me: as one wag put it, "it is any one who drinks more than you do!"

Up to the present time men have been affected more than women, at least to the extent that they can be identified – there is no doubt that heavy drinking does go on silently in the home and women have never been immune as witnessed by the sordid sketches of gin-drinking biddies a century or two ago. Experience varies with the practice of the physician; among the wives of top executives the problem is no light one.

Shakespeare gave us the seven ages of man; Dr. Max Glatt of the Alcoholic Addiction Unit has followed with the seven stages of alcoholic man:

1. Drunk at 20.
2. Amnesia or loss of memory attacks at 30.
3. Loss of control at 34.
4. Early morning drinking at 35.
5. Suicide contemplated at 36.
6. Medical advice for complications at 39.
7. The depths of a man's morale at 42.

The acceleration of the signs towards early middle life is striking and of course characteristic.

The divorced and widowed show a higher frequency than either single or married men; alcoholism may precede the one and follow the other. On the other hand it is married women who, until recent years, have shown a greater preponderance. The assumption by women of greater responsibility outside the home is beginning to take its toll among single and "career" women. There is no consistently clear relation of alcoholism to social class and this will soon be further blurred by the increasing affluence of living throughout social classes 1 to 5. Nevertheless, among those seeking help for their disorder, the social class 1, 2 and 3 (the social "middle" class) predominate, as might be expected, whether this help is from doctors or such organisations as Alcoholics Anonymous. The estimation of social class in the long-term alcoholic has been found to be difficult as the degeneracy of the individual may be accompanied by a pronounced fall in his social and occupational status.

This chapter is not a treatise on alcoholism but rather an attempt to present the problem in the light of its effects upon work and, at times, the effect of work upon the drinking pattern.

Those engaged in heavy labour, in hot conditions, requiring large fluid replacements such as foundrymen and miners, or those who belong to a select band of habit drinkers such as heavy transport drivers and meat, fruit and fish porters, publicans and seamen are especially at risk: it is the need for fluid replacement or the ready availability of alcohol which is one injurious factor, although it is possible that self-selection into the job may contribute to the higher frequency. Like so much of our understanding of today's illnesses, the potentiating or additive factors of a situation or environment are paramount: together with the basic inborn susceptibility, they push people beyond the point of return. For executives or others with the need to entertain for business or professional reasons, the possession of a "drinks cabinet", may appear to be a necessity. It should be resisted, because in the lives of all of us there come times when ease of access to a drink could lead to habit and the sad descent to the seven stages of alcoholic man (or woman!)

Some industrial organisations are sufficiently aware of the problem to see both the need to identify their alcoholics and also to rehabilitate them while preserving their self-respect. To this end formal programmes for recognition, prevention and rehabilitation have been adopted – it must be admitted much more widely in the United States than in this country. The justification for such a programme can be higher productivity, less waste, less absenteeism and fewer accidents. One American company estimated their programme saved $80,000 a year. In a recent government review of industrial health and safety* not a word is mentioned of alcohol as a cause of accidents, principally because of the absence of reported evidence, not because the situation does not exist. In other countries with heavy and different drinking patterns, notably France, the frequency of works accidents is known to be high at the commencement of the day shift, and is related to the habit of early morning drinking so prevalent among the working people. The relevance of this experience to the accident pattern in Scotland has not yet been assessed but would bear looking into in view of the problem of heavy drinking in that country.

PREVALENCE OF ALCOHOLISM RATES PER 100,000 POPULATION AGED 20 OR MORE

Place	Year	Jellinek Method	Independent Assessor
FRANCE	1951	5,200	7,300
U.S.A.	1953	4,390	—
ONTARIO, CANADA	1961	2,460	2,375
DENMARK	1948	1,950	1,750
ENGLAND/WALES	1948 1960–63	1,100	865

Source: Alcoholism and Drug Research Foundation, Toronto, Canada. (Project No. 23.)

Up till now there have not been any figures which can be directly compared with those from England and Wales. We have to be content with hospital admission statistics which are dependent on many features of life in Scotland which do not necessarily apply to populations south of the border. We must therefore still rely on critical observation as Dr. Martin Whittet recently reminded us in a diverting yet perceptive lecture to the Society of Occupational Medicine: ". . . it was a gentleman named Bowditch in 1872 who formulated a cosmic law of alcoholism. He considered that the effects of alcohol on individuals and society became more pernicious (unlike car-driving) the further north one went from the equator"! Relative to France and the United States, England and Wales would not appear to have a problem, but what are not apparent from their figures are the attitudes of people towards seeking advice and the methods and accuracy of medical and social diagnosis. Even within countries themselves the frequency has been shown to vary widely in relation to these variables as again Dr. Whittet pointed out in relation to Scotland.

* *Safety and Health at Work*, Report of the Committee 1970–72. Chairman, Lord Robens. H.M.S.O.

The long-term recovery rate of those salved from the trash-bin of alcoholism through effective company-sponsored programmes can be as high as 65 per cent in people who accept treatment.

Treatment of the alcoholic in industry essentially begins with the establishment of a declared company policy which is made known to each worker: the health education aspects are publicised, particularly the benefit to the individual of early consultation both in restoring his health and retaining his job. Whether the programme is administered through a company medical department or its consultant advisers will depend on several factors but will not affect the general outcome so long as it has the full support of the patient, his general practitioner and his close fellow-workers. The success of treatment depends largely upon the co-operation of all levels of management; they must be prepared to support him; without this he stands little chance. Thus the ethical problem of privileged information has to be considered and the agreement of the patient obtained as an essential prerequisite: details concern no one but patient and doctor – attitudes and rehabilitation concern all who work with the victim.

Treatment may be refused or be unsuccessful: at this time a decision will have to be made to end a man's employment, with the appropriate sickness benefits differing in no way from the system operating in other serious and progressive illnesses.

11 Respiratory Disease in Industry

Long before any industrial dust or fume can be incriminated to account for his respiratory illnesses, the inspired air of the average British workman is already polluted by the cloud of smoke drifting up from the cigarette habitually held in his mouth.

By closing your eyes and conjuring up an attractive meal you can set your salivary glands working overtime to whet your appetite. By the same mechanism you can soon sour your stomach, if you are sensitive enough, by imagining yourself in the saloon bar of a pub or the smoking section of a bus or train – before long you will hear the racking, bubbling exhausting cough of the man with chronic bronchitis or "the English disease".

The end result of breathing smoke-laden air which itself creates conditions for acute and later chronic destruction of the different parts of the breathing system, is the largest single cause of our enormous sickness absenteeism from industry. In the past, legislation has followed the identification of sources of industrial air pollution, and provided monetary compensation for those found to have suffered permanently. Until recently the harmful effects of cigarette smoking had not made the major league, but today we have all the evidence to confirm our previous suspicions that diseases of the respiratory tract and the heart are closely concerned with the inhaled products of combustion of cigarettes, whether factory made or "roll-your-own". Control of industrial pollution at the worksite is the responsibility of management, and the Factories Acts, Agricultural Acts, Offices, Shops & Railway Premises Act; all have the statutory powers to penalise those responsible if dangerous conditions arise. This is as it should be, but now that we know that the

84

additive effects of cigarette smoking will increase the damaging effects of air pollution, it is time that the personal responsibility of the working man or woman was called upon to control and ultimately rid the country of this wasteful problem.

Respiratory disease in industry is as old as man himself. When he began to chip his flints to make weapons and tools he found himself breathing fine quartz dust, in the same way as occurred until recently among the "flint-knappers" of East Anglia. The earliest books written about industrial disease, some over four hundred years ago, describe the occupations and causes of disease in those whose life expectancy was shortened. Skilled men in the mines were not easy to come by and their health and retention at work were considerations even then.

TABLE I

The environment	The physical nature of the pollutant	The condition of the soil
Heat, humidity	Animal, vegetable or	The normality of the
Air velocity	mineral	individual's defence
Electro-static forces	Solubility, size	processes
Dust	Concentration, ability to	Anatomical and physiological
Fume	sensitise body tissues	structure
		Length of exposure
Gas	Capacity for excretion	Total or dose weight of the
Aerosol	from body	damaging agent
	Cumulative effects	Habits of the person involved
	Stimulus of common	Their effects upon his resist-
	infectious agents to	ance reduced by exhaus-
	produce disease	tion, nutrition, smoking
		and alcohol

Social and industrial enactments over the past hundred years, coupled with the new methods of studying patterns of disease and scientific laboratory investigation, have enabled us to define, clarify and begin to take preventive measures against industrial respiratory disease.

The respiratory tract can be divided into upper, middle and lower, meaning consecutively the mouth, nose and back of the throat, then the single wind-pipe or trachea together with the twin main bronchial tubes, and finally the smaller bronchial tubes and lungs. When study of industrial respiratory disease began seriously, it was provoked by the ill-effects of the dust experienced in tunnelling, quarrying and mining coal, iron, gold, tin and the many forms of rock, the most important among them being quartz. But today, with new processes in the engineering, plastics and textile industries, with

G

silage gases, insecticides and sensitivity to fungi in agriculture, and in a host of other industries such as food processing and detergents where biologically active additives are introduced, industrial air pollution continues to create problems in all three parts of the respiratory tract (Table 2).

TABLE 2

Lung condition	Associated industrial cause when exposure is known
Acute pneumonia	Manganese, beryllium, cadmium vanadium, mouldy hay, degraded plastics
Asthma	Wood, feathers, wool, toluene di-isocyanates, platinum, vanadium
Chronic bronchitis	Cotton, flax, any dust or fume
Chronic fibrosis (shrinking of lung)	Free silica, coal, asbestos, talc, mica, bauxite, beryllium
X-ray deposition only	Iron, tin, barium

Gradually there has developed a better understanding of how respiratory disease affects the capacity of the worker. Many suffer short episodes which contribute to high sickness absenteeism; others have more lengthy illnesses due to chronic and increasingly disabling disease; some develop cancer.

If we accept that a reasonable life span continues to be the "three-score years and ten", then there remains a lot to be done to prevent productive men and women in the prime of life developing chronic bronchitis, pulmonary fibrosis, and cancer of the nose, throat, lung and its coverings; in addition to this there is the need to avoid the misery which these diseases bring with them to the actual process of dying.

With old processes being modified and new ones being constantly developed, those responsible must assure the operatives before a production line is set up, that any potential hazard will have been eliminated or at least contained. The sharing of this knowledge in a sensible way with the workers will go far in achieving their acceptance and co-operation in methods of good disease prevention.

The nose, mouth and throat, the intakes and exhausts of the respiratory system, have a very thin layer of baffling along the walls. This baffling consists of a few coarse hairs in the nose, but is mostly made up of a sticky layer of mucous which catches larger particles in the air. These are then ejected by blowing the nose or spitting; they may, however, be swallowed. The trachea and bronchial tubes have, in addition to the sticky mucous, very fine waving hairs called cilia which assist in propelling trapped particles away from the depths of the respiratory tract. These tubes, or the lower parts of them, are contractile and when irritated will close down to prevent damaging agents going deeper into the lung. With the reflex closing of the vocal chords in the larynx due to irritation anywhere along the tract, and their subsequent explosive opening, a cough occurs because of the pressure build-up in the lungs below by the muscles of the chest wall and diaphragm. But if the tubes only partially close they give rise to short-lived or more prolonged obstruction which, while it stops air going into the lungs, also traps it there and prevents it coming out; these are asthmatic symptoms, characterised by wheezing. Often a ball-valve effect arises from plugs of mucous secretion: air builds up in the cavities of the lungs which then expand so that the surface for gas exchange, made up of dozens of little lace-like air sacs, breaks down and is reduced in total area, thus diminishing exchange of oxygen and carbon dioxide. This is called emphysema and is a natural consequence of chronic bronchitis. This latter actually means a considerable excess of infected mucous secretion coupled with spasm of, and obstruction by, the bronchial tubes, leading to destruction of lung tissue.

At the very end of the line, at the gas exchange surface in the lung, a number of irritating agents cause local inflammation, swelling and inhibition of gaseous exchange. The reduction of oxygen in blood and tissues and build-up of carbon dioxide is very similar to the end results of chronic bronchitis and emphysema, but is not necessarily accompanied or preceded by them as the irritant and damaging action is too rapid and localised.

The result of all this is in the first place a lessening of the ability of affected people to work, and ultimately difficulty in finding the necessary energy even to exist. A dreadful vicious circle develops when the muscular efforts to breathe create a greater demand for oxygen than can be supplied by the obstructed lungs. The plight of these sufferers is terrible. But it is the sequence of symptoms, the morning cough with yellow phlegm, the slight wheezing or shortness of breath on moderate exercise, the recurring episodes of short illness, gradually lengthening, the "winter bronchitis", the bluish colour of the skin, lips and nail beds, the tug of the lower jaw with each breath while at rest, and the retching, bubbling, exhausting cough which creates the picture of chronic disabling respiratory disease. Some of it is preventable by the employer, but a lot of it is preventable by the individual, provided he is given sufficient health education and inducement.

SMOKERS LIKELIER VICTIMS

Bear in mind that this saga of events is overwhelmingly more likely to happen with cigarette smokers than non-smokers whether or not they have been exposed to industrial pollutant. Thus the first and most important element of both prevention and recognition is to persuade people to stop smoking. The day has not yet come when cigarette advertising is banned and other methods of dissuasion introduced, but we must act now, for we know that smoking itself will reduce the measurable lung function even before the additive effects of secondary bronchitis and emphysema, known together as obstructive broncho-pulmonary disease, appear. Once this happens the situation is irreversible.

12 Occupational Cancer Risks

Cancer is an emotive word: possibly its seeds are already within us but the spur to their growth, coming as it apparently does from many sources, may never occur during an average lifetime. We know very little about these sources; in an earlier chapter (5) the question of trigger mechanisms activating latent disease was briefly touched upon. Some clues to these mechanisms have emerged in the basic nature and the manner of action of certain agents, biological, chemical and mineral, which are definitely associated with the uncontrolled growth of cancer cells of a specific type and often localised in a particular organ, as for example the aromatic amine β-naphthylamine and the urinary tract. Our discussion will be restricted to this comparatively narrow though steadily widening field in what otherwise remains an enormous uncharted desert. Within this field the occupational cancer-producing agents occupy the major part and their proven relevance to cancer continues to provoke us to search for those other agents which exist in our every-day environment; these could be responsible for what has become the second leading cause of deaths in all age groups in this country. At this point, it is worth emphasising the strong probability that occupational and non-occupational influences activate and poten-tiate each other.

Whether all cancers arise from sleeping cancer cells either as a result of a provocation or, on the contrary, are released from restraint by the removal of naturally occurring substances such as circulating hormones, is beyond our present consideration: there is certainly good evidence that this mechanism operates in certain common cancers. On the other hand, particularly with skin cancer, there is no doubt that continued application of a cancer-provoking agent will cause the final appearance of malignant cells after a period of gradual change of the normal skin through various transitional stages. The scientists continue to wrestle with the problem.

Cancer arising from occupational exposure may come to light only after many years and for a variety of reasons the occupational significance may not at first be appreciated; the time span of a person's working life, the sequence and nature of jobs, the awareness of the physician, all play their part. So often, for many years before the appearance of the cancer, the patient may have been engaged in a non-hazardous occupation and forgotten or never known the implications of his earlier employment.

The diagnosis of cancer of the internal organs during life had to await the advent of reliable and safe investigative procedures; surgery coupled with effective pathological techniques only developed towards the end of last century. In contrast, cancer of the coverings of the body, the skin and modified skin lining the orifices, has been observed, described and treated for many centuries. Cancer is not a single entity having identical characteristics in all the various body tissues in which it arises: it is a term used loosely by laymen and doctor alike to describe a multitude of uncontrolled cell growths which, by size, shape and relation to surrounding structures, can displace, erode and alter the functions of healthy organs. In some instances the cancer may usurp normal physiological function and overproduce secretions which can themselves upset the body's usual metabolism: particular examples of these are certain types of cancer of the lung, thyroid and kidney, as far as it is known, unrelated to occupation.

Historically it was Percival Pott, surgeon to St. Bartholomew's Hospital in the City of London, who, in 1775 laid the corner-stone of our knowledge of the relation between a man's work and the development of cancer. In itself Pott's paper, on the cancer of the scrotum of chimney-sweeps, was of comparatively small significance when life expectancy was still abysmally low. But a hundred years later, when this began to increase, the causes of death were to move away from the accidents and infectious diseases towards the cancers and degenerative conditions. Pott's clinical observations were the first of their kind to be scientifically and methodically reported, but examination of several older descriptions of disease reveal that a relation between occupation and fatal disease was known to exist. The classical story of the lung disease of miners in the Schneeburg silver mines in southern Germany in the Middle Ages illustrates this well: they did in fact develop cancer of the lung, at the time known only as *mala metallorum*, almost certainly as a result of exposure to the ionising radiation coming from the bedrock.

Occupational cancer lends itself particularly to epidemiological, geographical and demographical studies because of the locality of certain industries and the nature of the population which may be exposed. The composition of a work-force will vary from industry to industry not only in age and sex but today also in national and racial make-up. On the whole people who develop occupational cancer tend to be younger than those in the general population who develop a similar disease but of unknown cause. The *National Atlas of Disease Mortality in the United Kingdom*, compiled by Professor Melvyn Howe, has already pointed to the remarkable regional variations in cancer mortality, and while the occupational factors have not as yet been separately identified they may well be responsible for a significant part of the overall picture.

What are these cancer-provoking factors and from what processes do they arise? First and broadly the injurious effects on the body, apart from being nearly always unconscionably slow, can sometimes be preceded by overt "pre-cancerous" changes in the tissues. These may affect skin or internal organs and this recognition serves on which to base a crude classification of occupational cancer. Secondly the processes themselves: the cancer-provoking irritant stimulus may arise from the natural elements, such as ultra-violet or ionising radiation, the first particularly in those pale-skinned people continually exposed over many years, sailors and farmers, and surveyors in tropical countries. Chronic friction has been a noted factor in skin cancer associated with soot and dirt. It is said that the cattle herders of Mexico have been particularly prone to develop cancer of the scrotum due to the constant friction of the high pommel of their saddle and soiled and rough clothing. The production of raw materials and manufacture of refined goods whether in one stage or through many complicated processes remains the principal danger today.

The handling of cancer-provoking materials is now much better appreciated in industry although less so in the laboratory and in the home among "do-it-yourself" enthusiasts: only in industry do statutory regulations apply in a meaningful manner. A great deal of health education is provided however by manufacturing associations concentrating on the most commonly used materials. The materials most prolific in their effects are pitch, tars and various kinds of mineral oils. Exposure to them, being an everyday occurrence in some workers, is undoubtedly dose related: this is particularly the case in road construction, manufacture of sealing materials and the multitude of uses to which mineral oils are put. The carcinogenicity or cancer-producing activity of coal-tar, shale-oil and crude petroleum products depends upon the nature of the hydrocarbon fractions they contain: mineral oils, through denaturing processes such as heating and bacterial contamination or the presence of additives and impurities, will provoke cancer. Oils which have been prepared for certain types of textile machinery and the special oils used in the cutting of metal by automatic lathes have been notorious in the past. Such dangerous processes should by now have been eliminated in this country, but the late effects on men and occasionally women who were exposed many years ago may still be seen. Thus it is so important that personal cleanliness, constant surveillance and medical examination be continued even beyond retirement. Such a programme has in fact been carried out for a number of years through the laboratory facilities provided by the Rubber Industries Manufacturers Association, following the tragic consequences of cancer of the urinary tract developing in workers exposed, before 1949, to the antioxidant β-naphthylamine. The time interval before any evidence of cancer arises may be as much as thirty years: those people who worked in the production departments of the rubber industry before 1950 have been offered regular examination of their urine, which, by special techniques, can indicate at an early stage the presence of cancer. This is done with the hope that immediate treatment can deal with the disease at a treatable stage. The establishment of this scheme has been nation-wide, costly but productive in that although many workers have indeed developed cancer this has been detected at an early stage. The substitution of dangerous substances has been a long and expensive business but must be seen to have been done in our now enlightened society. Still one of the most disturbing features in the war against this kind of disease has been the failure of people, the workers themselves, the employers and the doctors to realise the relation of cancer to occupation and to follow this up by notification to the authorities under the statutory obligations. Only in this way can the disease be recognised and eliminated.

It is fair to say that there remains considerable doubt as to the full extent of the problem and this may be especially true of those other forms of cancer which arise in the deeper tissues of the body. I do not think any useful purpose will be served by discussing these in detail but rather to indicate broadly the fields in which they arise and the nature of their activity. To complement this there are several admirable reference books where much fuller information is available.

The accompanying table is by no means all-inclusive but does give some idea of the size and nature of the problem. New materials are constantly being produced and many are now subjected to cancer tests analagous to those in the pharmaceutical industry: nevertheless, this is not a requirement of every new material but rather

TABLE I

Proven carcinogen	Mode of entry to body	Site of cancer	Industrial process

COAL TAR
  Soot, Pitch
  Tar, Creosote
SHALE OILS
PETROLEUM
  Cutting oils
  Polycylic
  hydrocarbons
	Surface
	contamination
		SKIN
		Face, hands,
		arms
		scrotum
			Fractionisation of
			of coal, shale and
			petroleum: use of
			products.

PHYSICAL IRRITANTS
  Ultra-violet rays
  Ionising radiation
  Friction
  Local heat
	Surface conta-
	mination:
	Inhalation of
	irradiated dust
		Skin
		Lungs
		Blood
		Bones
			Sun exposure
			(U.V.R.)
			Handling during
			radioactive pro-
			processes and sub-
			stances.
			Mining of uranium,
			haematite, fluorspar.

METALS AND
MINERALS
  Arsenic
  Chromium
  Nickel
  Asbestos
	Surface
	contamination:
	Inhalation of
	fume
		Skin, mucous
		membranes
		Naso-pharynx
		Lungs
			Production, use of/
			and accidental
			contamination with

CHEMICALS AND
DYES
  β-Naphthylamine
  Benzidine
  Auramine
  Magenta
	Absorption
	through skin
		Genito-urinary
		tract
			Manufacture,
			Use of

ISOPROPYL ALCOHOL	Inhalation	Naso-pharynx	Manufacture (dis- continued) process

depends on the known or potential carcinogenic activity of the chemical "family" from which the material is derived or into which it falls. The time-lag before suspicious tissue changes are seen varies greatly: even in the final analysis the extrapolation of animal results to humans must leave some doubt.

One final note of warning: as in other forms of disease, the potentiation of one substance by another or the additive effects of several substances being more dangerous than the sum of the effect of each one individually are now clearly of great significance. Nowhere perhaps is this more impressive than in Selikoff's work on

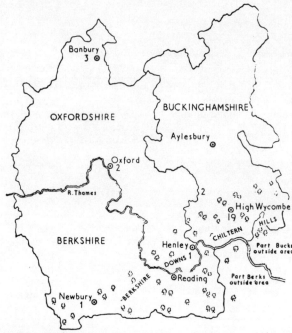

Fig. 18 Map of area showing numbers of cases of adenocarcinoma ascertained in persons ever employed in the furniture industry according to place of exposure. (*From "Nasal Cancer in Woodworkers in the Furniture Industry" Acheson, E. D. et al. Brit. Med. Jour. 2. 587–596. 1968*).

the effects of smoking in asbestos workers: he was able to show conclusively that those who smoke cigarettes and have been occupationally exposed to asbestos dust have eight times the chance of developing lung cancer as compared to those smokers who were not asbestos workers; furthermore, they had one hundred times the chance of cancer compared to those who neither smoked nor were exposed to asbestos!

Before closing this chapter, an example of the fascinating detection work involved in the recognition of an occupational cancer problem is worth illustrating, coming as it does from an unexpected source, set in an attractive part of southern England. In the early 1960s it became apparent to an observant surgeon that a significant proportion of the patients that she was treating for cancer of the nasal cavities lived and worked in the town of High Wycombe in Buckinghamshire. Furthermore, they worked almost exclusively in the furniture-making trade and were on the whole relatively younger than people elsewhere who developed the same somewhat rare disease. Through the facilities of the Oxford cancer registry covering the adjoining counties of Oxfordshire, Buckinghamshire and Berkshire it was confirmed that there was an unexplained concentration of patients with cancer of the nasal cavities in the High Wycombe area. Now High Wycombe is an ancient town which lies in a fold of the chalky Chiltern Hills, along the banks of the River Wye in the county of Buckinghamshire. It is 28 miles north-west of London and is an example of a dispersed industrial town with a population approaching 60,000, set in the midst of attractive agricultural country, mixed arable, dairy and livestock farming. The local industries consist of engineering, chemicals and printing, with furniture manufacturing predominating. There are today nearly 2,000 cabinet- and chair-makers in High Wycombe, the largest concentration in the country, virtually half that of the cabinet- and chair-makers in the whole country. High Wycombe has traditionally made furniture from beech trees which grow well on chalky soil, and in the second half of the eighteenth century chair-making was a thriving industry. Within the last sixty years not only have imported hardwoods taken the place of beech but the industry has spread elsewhere locally to Oxford and Banbury. However, in High Wycombe in 1939 there were 150 small firms with 5,000 workers which together turned out one and a half million wooden chairs annually: at that time factory conditions varied enormously, particularly in the provision of exhaust ventilation and removal of wood dust. The total number of local furniture workers has now fallen and the number of factories has also decreased although those remaining have larger premises and much improved conditions.

The original investigation in the 1960s revealed that woodworkers in the local furniture industries had an annual average incidence of adenocarcinoma (a glandular form of cancer) of the nasal cavities seven times greater than those people in all local occupations together and, more startlingly, one thousand times more than the figures for the general population in the rest of the country! Early in the present decade it was found that people elsewhere in England and Wales who had worked in the furniture industry also bore an increased risk of this type of cancer: interestingly, two other groups who had been exposed to dusts of biological origin, boot and shoe makers and repairers and women in cotton textile plants were also found to be more at risk, although the latter group require further study before any definite conclusions can be drawn.

I have reproduced a table from this unique report which clearly shows the different occupations among the patients whose records were examined and the predominance among wood and leather workers. The occupational histories of two patients may bring home better than any bare descriptions of working conditions what it is that workers in this trade have had to contend with, certainly until very recently. Perhaps it would be too optimistic to hope that no

TABLE 2

CASES AND CONTROLS, INCLUDING RETIRED PERSONS, DISTRIBUTED BY OCCUPATIONAL ORDER (MALES ONLY)

	Occupational order	Adenocarcinomas			Controls	
		At diagnosis or on retirement*	Main occupation*	Expected numbers	At diagnosis or on retirement	Main occupation
I	Farmers, foresters, and fishermen	3	2	4·2	6	6
II	Miners and quarrymen	3	3	2·7	4	4
III	Gas, coke, and chemicals makers	1	2	0·6	2	2
IV	Glass and ceramics makers	1	1	0·3	0	0
V	Furnace, forge, etc. workers	3	3	1·3	0	1
VI	Electrical and electronic workers	1	1	2·2	2	1
VII	Engineers and allied trade workers	5	5	11·2	9	9
VIII	Woodworkers	24	28	2·1	8	9
	Furniture industry†	15	19	0·2	4	5
	Others and unspecified	9	9	1·9	4	4
IX	Leather workers	7	7	0·5	1	1
X	Textile workers	2	2	0·8	2	2
XI	Clothing workers	2	2	0·5	0	0
XII	Food, drink, and tobacco workers	1	1	1·4	1	1
XIII	Paper and printing workers	0	0	1·1	1	1
XIV	Makers of other products	0	0	0·9	1	1
XV	Construction workers	1	1	2·7	4	4
XVI	Painters and decorators	1	1	1·6	2	2
XVII	Drivers of cranes, etc.	0	0	1·5	1	1
XVIII	Labourers, n.e.c.	3	3	6·1	5	5
XIX	Transport and communication workers	1	1	6·7	12	12
XX	Warehousemen, etc.	2	0	2·6	2	2
XXI	Clerical workers	2	2	5·7	2	2
XXII	Sales workers	3	2	6·3	6	6
XXIII	Service, sport, and n.e.c. workers	6	5	4·1	6	5
XXIV	Administrators and managers	2	2	3·1	1	1
XXV	Professional technical workers	4	4	6·0	6	7
XXVI	Armed forces	0	0	1·5	1	0
XXVII	Inadequately described	2	2	2·2	0	0
	Total	80	80	80	85	85

* The cases are shown by occupation (a) at diagnosis or on retirement and (b) main occupation.

† It has been assumed that all the persons enumerated at the census in occupational category 081, and about half those in category 082, were working in the furniture industry.

increase in this kind of cancer will occur in the future, but the fact remains that for the time being the outbreak seems to have reached its peak before 1965.

Case 002. Entered the furniture industry in 1917 as an apprentice cabinet-maker. The whole of his working life was spent in the furniture industry in Oxford. From 1917 to 1929 he made sectional book-cases, principally out of American oak. From 1929 to the beginning of his illness in 1962 he worked for a small firm making school and educational furniture for which the principal woods were American and Austrian oak, Parana pine, Douglas fir, Spanish chestnut, Cyprus pine and a very small quantity of beech. According to his sister-in-law, with whom he lived, he used to come home at night covered with dust. He was never exposed to smoke, and was not a snuff-taker.

Case 007. He started work in 1918 as an apprentice cabinet-maker and worked in a number of different firms in the trade in High Wycombe. Before the war he was exposed to mahogany, oak and a certain amount of beech. He always worked in the cabinet-making shop, never on chairs. He also suffered from "mahogany colds" (exposure to certain kinds of mahogany can cause an acute rhinitis or head cold). According to his wife his underclothes were often pink with sawdust. He never took snuff.

The nature of the substance or substances in wood dust which may be responsible for initiating the painful and malignant disease of nasal cancer still eludes us. It seems they were certainly present in 1920 and persisted until as recently as 1940, because no patient has presented with the disease who commenced work since that year. Nevertheless, some or all of the substances may still be present, for the development of cancerous changes may take many years. Wood dusts are notorious in causing both acute bronchial allergy (asthma) and dermatitis.

The known components of wood dust are the wood itself, its resins, silicon dioxide (silica), glues, insecticides and fungicides with which it may have been treated. It is unlikely that varnish and lacquers are responsible because the use of these does not figure in the occupational picture and people using these materials exclusively do not present any unusual frequency of the cancer. It is known that certain other substances will cause nasal cancer, among them the metal nickel, isopropyl alcohol and radium. The position of snuff is indeterminate but may once have been an additive factor. We are not yet in a position to even guess at what is the specific agent: nevertheless, one avenue of approach may be worth pursuing, that of the metal content of certain woods. Workers in other fields have been analysing certain trees for some years now and using the metal profiles to assist in finding underlying ore bodies. Tree wood may selectively accumulate metals, in particular arsenic, lead and mercury. To show that there is "nothing new under the sun" it should be recalled that the ancient craft of lead glazing of pottery was carried out thousands of years ago by using the silica and lead content of the ash of ash trees as the source of the vitreous material: indeed this method is still pursued by certain specialist potters. I do not know the metal content of beech trees, but plants reduced to their ash may contain metals in the following amounts:

TABLE 3

Copper	50– 150	parts per million
Zinc	500–2,000	,, ,, ,,
Lead	25– 75	,, ,, ,,
Molybdenum	10– 70	,, ,, ,,
Nickel	5– 100	,, ,, ,,
Manganese	20–1,000	,, ,, ,,

TABLE 4

SOME VALUES FOR INDIVIDUAL WESTERN CANADIAN TREES ARE ALSO OF INTEREST

2nd Year	Copper	Zinc	*Parts per million* Molybdenum	Lead
Mountain balsam	64	3,500	86	260
Douglas fir	400	6,800	43	640
Engelmann spruce	120	3,600	17	130
Limber pine (*Pinus flexilis*)	270	4,400	26	190
Red cedar (*Thuja plicata*)	288	4,300	15	290
Alder (*Alnus sp.*)	280	7,100	34	410
Willow (*Salix sp.*)	150	11,000	16	490

It should in fairness be said that the idea that metal in plants might in some way be injurious to human beings is no more than speculation and awaits further research.

I hope therefore that this description of cancer of the naso-pharynx in the furniture industry has helped to give you an idea of the complexity and intricacy of some occupational health problems.

13 Metals and our Bodies

Today's doctors have been taught their science and learnt their art by manual, visual and empirical testing, aided by epidemiological experience; in achieving an ever-increasing degree of success their diagnostic acumen has required laboratory technology to support it, though not necessarily to control it. The almost universal requirement has been the presence of symptomatic and overt disease, the end result rather than the earliest beginnings of a pathological process. Today it is no longer justifiable on humanitarian, sociological or economic grounds to wait for symptomatic disease to arise; procedures which are now available should be employed to anticipate and prevent disease provided they are reasonably accurate, reproducible, acceptable to the recipient (for he is not yet a patient), and relatively inexpensive.

Current techniques can, *inter alia*, obtain presymptomatic information useful in screening for the absorption of certain metals, biological agents and chemical compounds. They consist either of the direct measurement of body load and excretion or the indirect measurement of effects through enzyme and metabolic distortion and the excretion of breakdown or intermediate products. Jager has expressed this clearly:

"The objective must be the detection, in an early preclinical stage, of biological responses of the body to potentially dangerous materials. The detection of these responses in a preclinical, reversible and non-incapacitating stage, allows the prevention of non-acceptable biological responses and progressive development of occupational disease with subjective manifestations, "complaints", and, finally, actual symptoms of disease. Actual disease is one of the last phases and a late result of a series of disturbances

99

and compensations, which occur as an interaction between the body and a toxicant . . . adequate preventive measures can be taken only if we know the dose response relationship which exists between, on the one hand, the toxicant, which must include the exposure over long or short periods as well as the pre-existing body-burden and, on the other hand, the effect of this dose on the subject."

He goes on to quote Hatch

"To establish a basic scale of dose requires that the critical site of intoxication be known and that the mechanism of damaging action be understood in such fundamental terms as to distinguish clearly between the nature of the active agent operating at the critical site and the form of the external agent."

Sufficient information has accumulated to suggest that the influence of minute amounts of certain substances, for example the "trace metals", either from deprivation or excess, upon the metabolism of animals and man, can lead to severe metabolic disorders including disturbances of growth, the quickening of degenerative processes and cancer-producing effects. Perhaps the earliest relevant illustration of such influence was the demonstration of the selective growth factor or metal dependence by which Raulin showed that the common fungus, Aspergillus, required the presence of zinc for adequate growth: that was over a hundred years ago.

Today there is an imposing list of conditions which have been shown, in man, to be related in some way to metals. One of the most dramatic examples has been the appearance and subsequent disappearance over the first fifty years of this century of Pink disease, which describes the colour of the extremities of children and is related to the absorption of mercury from teething powders in those peculiarly susceptible. We know that many physiological processes are regulated by metal-dependent enzymes, and are aware that the possibility of molecular substitution by trace metals, by interfering with the enzyme catalytic reactions, could be a major pathway to disease. During the process of evolution this phenomenon has been under stress for the respiratory pigments of plants and some animals may utilise different metals, presumably in the process of adaptation to changing sources and requirements in the course of species survival.

With increasing sophistication of analysis and the interest and awareness of investigators, the relation between trace metals and some common disorders is becoming apparent, whether in association or as cause or effect. The advent of long-term renal dialysis (artificial kidney) has introduced the risk of increasing or reducing trace metals beyond their useful threshold by the use of water supplies which may contain varying amounts of these elements: these possibilities serve to illustrate the environmental sources which must be considered when anticipating or suspecting trace metal effects. The approach that should be made bears a close analogy to the Hippocratic concept of the means by which disease should be investigated – it has stood the test of time for nearly two and a half thousand years.

". . . Whoever wishes to investigate medicine properly should proceed thus – In the first place to consider the seasons of the year and what effect each of them produces (for they are not at all alike but differ much from themselves in regard to their changes). Then the wind, the hot and the cold such as are common to all countries and then such as are peculiar to each locality. We must also consider the qualities of the waters for as they differ from one another in taste and weight so also do they differ much more in their qualities. In the same manner when one comes to a city to which he is a stranger, he should consider its situation. How it lies as to the wind and the rising sun for its influence is not the same whether it lies to the North or the South, to the rising or to the setting sun. These things one should consider most attentively and concerning the waters which the inhabitants use whether they may be marshy or soft or hard and running from elevated and rocky situations, and then if saltish and unfit for cooking and the ground whether it be named and deficient in water or wooded and well watered and whether it lies in a hollow confined situation or if elevated and cold, and the mode in which the inhabitants live and what are their pursuits. Whether they are fond of drinking and eating to excess and given to indolence or are fond of exercise and labour and not given to excess in eating and drinking.

"From these things he must proceed to investigate everything else for if one knows all things well or at least the greater part of them he cannot miss knowing when he comes into a strange city either the diseases peculiar to the place or the particular nature of common diseases so that he will not be in doubt as to the treatment of the diseases or common mistakes as is likely to be the case provided one had not previously considered these matters. And in particular, as the seasons and the year advance he can tell what epidemic diseases will attack the city, either in summer or in winter, and what each individual will be in danger of experiencing from the changed regimen, for knowing the change of the seasons, the risings and settings of the stars, how each of them takes place, he will be able to know beforehand what sort of year is going to ensue. Having made

H

these investigations and knowing beforehand the seasons such a man must be acquainted with each bit and must succeed in the provision of health and would be by no means unsuccessful in the practice of his art, and if it shall be thought that these things belong rather to meteorology it will be admitted on second thought that astronomy contributes not a little but a very great deal indeed to medicine for with the seasons the digestive organs of man undergo a change. . . ."

Throughout this country and elsewhere screening programmes for selected trace elements are now being pursued, mainly in relation to biological monitoring of industrial processes, but also in certain geographical areas where suspected excesses or deficiencies exist due to geological and other causes. There is indeed a great need to achieve simple and inexpensive methods by which populations at risk can be monitored: at the same time, there is some justification, in view of our continuing ignorance of the causes of many symptomatic disorders, for attempting to screen populations for a variety of elements to which they may or may not be known to be environmentally or occupationally exposed and which might conceivably be affecting their health sufficiently for this to be examined, along with the traditional methods of questionnaire, attendance at the doctor's surgery, sickness absence from work, and mortality data. One particular group of people receiving very thorough monitoring of their mineral metabolism are the astronauts. The importance of negative mineral balances in future prolonged missions is self-evident. Like so much of the applied research in the space programmes the study of human metabolism may yield information of great importance for those of us who remain earthbound.

The potential for large screening programmes to generate a demand for extra health and sickness services is now better appreciated than at their inception, but a programme of the nature suggested is unlikely to do this: instead it could provide a range of "normal" levels within which people could safely continue their activities without fear of long-term ill effects. Existing advice to people is based either on relatively crude environmental levels of toxicants or conversely on too sensitive biological testing by procedures which fail to provide realistic data in terms of ill health without creating unjustified anxiety. Until now, techniques have not allowed population screening on a wide scale and "normal" (or usual) ranges have been derived from data on comparatively small groups often with a degree of bias provided by variable peculiarities of the population concerned, whether related to age, sex, method of selection, physical and biochemical characteristics or apparently unassociated environmental factors.

Who are we primarily concerned with in population screening?

This has, until now, dependeded upon the awareness of an association between cause and effect and these effects may in turn depend
upon the varying threshold sensitivities of different individuals:
rates of absorption and turnover in heavy manual workers due to
muscular work, heavy breathing and food and fluid consumption;
the peculiar sensitivity of the growing tissues of children; the possession of genetic traits by some populations which makes them
especially vulnerable; personal habits such as cigarette smoking,
now known to potentiate the effects of a variety of absorbed substances. To be meaningful in any screening programme, all these
and others beside must be identified and measured before conclusions
can be reached in regard to any single agent. The exponential
growth of a holistic approach soon becomes apparent; so we are
forced back to a reasonable compromise acceptable to the majority
of a population both in terms of recognisable effects and in terms of
economics. Criteria could be identified by which a few susceptible
people might be "screened out" of what is an acceptable risk to the
majority. It is in this area that research should be concentrated to
find rapid and reproducible tests to show the effects of a substance on
a representative group of individuals. We are long familiar with this
technique both in general medicine and in special industrial environments, for skin testing is among the most valuable of preventive as
well as diagnostic measures, whether for substances acting on the
skin or on the body tissues generally. Until now, the use of these
techniques for the prevention of disease in the general community
has been nearly always confined to biological preparations such as
bacterial, protozoal and metazoal extracts for the recognition of the
possession of antibody among special groups. In industry three
metals in particular may be tested for in this way, platinum, nickel
and beryllium, although the danger of producing a primary hyper-
sensitive effect from beryllium is recognised.

One of the most difficult problems is to keep a sense of balance
among all the mass of evidence that is now turning up, not all of it
scientific. For instance, the fact that substances are found in biological material does not necessarily prove their harmfulness, for
many plant and animal species have the ability to concentrate
certain substances far beyond their general level in the environment;
examples being lead and mercury in certain trees, the ash and spruce
respectively, and cadmium in shellfish. It is possible that this very
power of concentrating is one of nature's compensating and self-
cleansing mechanisms. The adaptability of some organisms is
remarkable and from this we should take heart for the future – the
story of certain moths of industrial England in the nineteenth
century with their colour change to match the industrially polluted

background is a case in point. Even children can handle relatively large amounts of lead and store it away in the bones. Providing no other insults, such as an unrelated illness, arise to precipitate the release of substances from bone, the lead remains apparently harmless. This is not to say that it should either be allowed to get there or remain there, but balance and judgement is required before summarily accepting that it and other substances are continuously harmful.

Metals are becoming increasingly implicated in the study of epidemiology patterns: some are vitally necessary to man, animals and plants for continual survival and good health. Others compete with and may substitute each other in enzymatic and metabolic processes. The sources of both desirable and undesirable metals are distributed through the liquids we drink, the food (whether of plant or animal origin) we eat, the air we breathe, the medicines that are prescribed for us and the material which may be absorbed through our skin and our lungs at work. Of all these, inhalation is probably the most important.

Up until very recently health workers have been restricted to considering overt disease occurring as a result of heavy intoxication, but current analytical methods enable us to anticipate gross disorder by concentrating attention at cell and enzyme level. It is fortunate that these methods have been developed just at the time when we have become aware of the overwhelming need to prevent recognisable illness in both humans and cattle from environmental pollution: it has been the veterinary workers who have had the advantage over us in realising the delicate balance that is maintained by a variety of trace metals in the food of meat and milk producing animals, particularly the ruminants. The emphasis that has failed to be placed on recognisable human disease associated with these elements contrasts with the awareness that we possess for the deviations due to the alkali metals Sodium (Na) and Potassium (K) (one electron in the outermost shell and exhibit a valence of 1), the alkaline earth metals Calcium (Ca) and Magnesium (Mg) (two outer electrons, valency of 2) and the transition element Iron (Fe) (high density, high melting and boiling points: forms alloys and absorbs gases; has a variable valency, Fe^2 (ferrous) and Fe^3 (ferric)). Chemical recognition of their presence and concentration has been relatively easy and has led to the appreciation of the essential nature of their alterations and effects within fairly narrow limits. But molecular biology has now introduced us to the phenomenon of trace metal dependence of enzymes concurrently with our growing awareness of the problems of chemical pollution of the general environment: until a few years ago our knowledge and interest was restricted to changes in the industrial environment, with their relatively short-term effects. The examples of beryllium, asbestos and the β-naph-thylamines in the rubber and chemical industries have served to alert us to the subtle and more serious long-term effects of low level chronic exposure on the general population (Table 1).

TABLE 1

THE RELATION OF CERTAIN METALS TO WELL-RECOGNISED HUMAN CLINICAL DISORDERS OR CONDITIONS

Metal	Some known or suspected clinical disorders or conditions associated with increased absorption	Sources of metal absorption	Conditions associated with a decrease in body levels
ARSENIC	Gastro-intestinal symptoms Thickening of skin Cancer of skin Peripheral nerve degeneration	Pesticides Industrial Pollution Medicine (seldom today)	Failure of growth
CADMIUM	High blood pressure Myocardial infarction Acute inflammation lung Nephritis (kidney inflammation) Skeleton deformities	Electroplating Smelting Smoking cigarettes Welding	
COBALT	Lung inflammation Myocarditis (heart) muscle inflamma-tion) Excessive red blood cell formation	Hard metal manufacture Additive to certain beers (now ceased)	Pernicious anaemia
CHROMIUM	Cancer of lung Ulcers of skin and lining of nose Myocardial infarction	Mining Electroplating Cement manufac-ture and use	
COPPER	Wilson's disease (liver and nervous system damage) Kidney degeneration Lathyrism – *L. sativos* – a kind of pea – a form of paralysis in the tropics	Soil Pesticide Smelting	Failure of hair to crimp Skin disorders

TABLE 1—(*continued*)

Metal	Some known or suspected clinical disorders or conditions associated with increased absorption	Sources of metal absorption	Conditions associated with a decrease in body levels
LEAD	Abdominal colic Convulsions Anaemia Muscle degeneration	Old paint Fumes from melting and smelting Antiknock agent in petrol	
MAGNESIUM			Collapse and convulsions in infancy
MERCURY	Neurosis ("mad-hatter syndrome") Inflammation of gums Tremors Nervous tissue degeneration Kidney inflammation	Switchgear Laboratories Dental surgeries Mining Smelting	
MANGANESE	Inflammation of lungs Parkinsonism (disorder of gait and coarse tremor)	Mining Smelting Welding	Certain disorders of immunity mechanisms
NICKEL	Skin disorder Cancer of lung Myocardial infarction	Electroplating Smelting Direct contact with metal	
VANADIUM	Green tongue and High blood cholesterol	Welding dust from oil-burning furnaces	
ZINC			Lung tuberculosis Women on Pill Pregnancy Skin ulcers Failure of wound healing Growth retardation Mongolism Kidney failure

As with chemical drugs, so can metals in a biological medium influence each other's activity and that of other nutrients. We have long recognised the reciprocal relationship of calcium and phosphorus, and calcium and lead; more recently of calcium and magnesium. Within the last few years interference with absorption and effects on the developing foetus have been demonstrated, as for instance when selenium can prevent the teratogenic effects of cadmium and arsenic, or the administration of large amounts of iron can reduce the absorption of manganese. Metal effects in the human body depend upon atomic weight, number, valency, solubility and ionisation. In addition a number of metals and elements are known to actively sensitise tissue cells.

Metabolism is the maintenance of a balanced state of growth and decay through the evolution of energy required for cell multiplication and function to produce kinetic and mental activity. The essential components of the myriads of biochemical reactions besides carbohydrates, fats and protein, consist of vitamins, the correct bacterial flora in the bowel and the necessary enzymes made up of amino-acids with their distinctive polypeptide chains of proteins, some of which at least require a trace of specific metal. Yet again, as we have seen, complex respiratory pigments in both vertebrates and invertebrates need the addition of metal to perform their vital function of energy transfer (Table 2). The role of the metallo-enzyme catalyst either in a laboratory test or in the body can be illustrated by carbonic anhydrase, an enzyme in red blood cells which accelerates the solution and evolution of carbon dioxide: this enzyme is dependent upon zinc and was one of the first to be identified.

TABLE 2

Respiratory pigments	Metal activator
Haemoglobin	Iron
Chlorophyll	Magnesium
	Manganese
Respiratory pigment of molluscs	Copper
Ditto of Sea-squirts	Vanadium

In the case of the metallo-dependent enzymes, which are widely distributed in nature and in our own bodies, the situation is complex. Enzymes are proteins, complex interlocking amino-acids, possessing specific spatial orientation of chemical constituents. This allows the enzyme molecule to fit that of the substrate upon which it acts. It may consist of several components – iso-enzymes – each of which still act in the same substrate. Foreign, toxic substrates do not possess these precise spatial requirements as do natural foodstuffs; thus only incomplete metabolisation occurs. Enzymes have additional needs in that they require co-factors or activators, metals and/or vitamins: anything that will inactivate them will render the enzyme inert – e.g. beryllium, cyanide, lead, mercury, arsenic: competition or more correctly molecular substitution is the mechanism involved (Table 3).

TABLE 3

SOME WELL-KNOWN ENZYMES IN THE HUMAN BODY – SELECTED FROM OVER 200 ENZYMES

	Listed by Davies (Ref.), metal is active part of prosthetic group or incorporated in enzyme itself
Alcohol dehydrogenase (liver)	Zinc
Alkaline phosphatase	Zinc
Arginase	Cadmium Manganese
Ascorbic acid	Copper
Carbonic anhydrase	Zinc
Ceruloplasmin	Copper
Choline esterase	Calcium
Creatin kinase	Magnesium
Desoxyribonuclease	Magnesium Manganese
Lactate dehydrogenase	Iron
Phosphorylase	Magnesium
Pyruvate kinase	Potassium
	Magnesium
	Ammonium
	Rubidium (Rb)
Succinate dehydrogenase	Iron
Xanthine oxidase	Iron
	Molybdenum

Davies, I. J. T. *The Clinical Significance of the Essential Biological Metals.* London, 1972, p. 126.

Human biochemical individuality has been observed since Garrod's original observations on the "inborn errors of metabolism" in 1908: before and following this many doctors were brought up to recognise a constitutional predisposition to disease – a diathesis: the explanation of this phenomenon eluded us until the recognition and measurement of enzymatic differences became feasible. The genetic basis has been established and the frequency of biochemical individuality is now reckoned to be significant. The accompanying table devised by Prof. Harris of University College, London, illustrates the complexity of these "errors" and the extent to which they have been investigated (Table 4), yet there is no evidence that any of these conditions is closely related to metal dependency though one suspects most of them have not been investigated from this viewpoint.

So far, we may accept Prasad's and other's view that most trace elements function through their association with enzymes and other proteins, nucleic acids and macromolecules. We have been aware for some time that alterations in plasma proteins will effect the concentration of calcium, iron and magnesium. There is evidence that other metals, notably zinc, chromium, nickel and manganese, are intimately related to protein synthesis and turnover, and their measurement and deviation from the assumed "normal" levels observed in such varying conditions as are listed in Table 1. Certain immunity mechanisms in the blood may apparently be inhibited by manganese and patients have been said to improve when given this metal. A rich source of manganese is tea!

A trace metal which has occasioned considerable interest recently is zinc. It has a suspected role in protein desoxyribose nucleic acid and ribose nucleic acid synthesis, a use to which it has once again been put in treating surgical wounds, decubitus and other indolent ulcers: it was an empirical remedy as "red lotion" (zinc sulphate) and zinc oxide three generations ago! Platelets and red blood cells are relatively rich in zinc and a large molecular protein has been found to have a zinc content of $400-700\mu$ G per g (G) – this could be a specific zinc building protein analagous to the specific transfer proteins for iron and copper. That metals are easily bound to protein we already know in the case of the above and calcium, levels for which in the blood have to be adjusted in relation to the main fraction of serum protein (albumin). Interestingly the presence of a high phytate content of the diet reduces the availability of zinc as well as calcium: phytates are higher in coarsely milled grain, a frequent constituent of "natural" foods and unleavened bread and chupattys, a favourite food of Indian immigrants. The phenomenon of industrial "metal fume fever" due to inhalation of zinc and copper fumes is an example of metallo-protein hypersensitivity, already shown to be a serious risk in some people exposed to beryllium. We have of course been long familiar with the zinc binding power of fish-roe protein used in the manufacture of Protamine-zinc Insulin. Zinc's role in low protein calorie malnutrition states both in undeveloped countries and among debilitated young and old in the United States is currently under study.

Industrial metal pollutants cover almost the whole gamut of the elements; many of these are discharged into the atmosphere or disappear down the sewers to reappear in our water; only a pro-

TABLE 4

ENZYMES WHICH HAVE BEEN SHOWN TO BE DEFICIENT IN VARIOUS "INBORN ERRORS OF METABOLISM"

Disorders of carbohydrate metabolism

 1. hexokinase (Congenital haemolytic disease)
 2. triosephosphate isomerase (Congenital haemolytic disease)
 3. phosphohexose isomerase (Congenital haemolytic disease)
 4. pyruvate kinase (Congenital haemolytic disease)
 5. 2.3 diphosphoglycerate mutase (Congenital haemolytic disease)
 6. phosphoglycerate kinase (Congenital haemolytic disease)
 7. glucose-6-phosphate dehydrogenase (Favism; primaquine sensitivity; congenital haemolytic anaemia)
 8. glucose-6-phosphatase (Glycogen disease, type I)
 9. amylo (1,4) glucosidase (Glycogen disease, type II)
10. amylo (1,6) glucosidase (Glycogen disease, type III)
11. amylo (1,4→1,6) transglucosidase (Glycogen disease, type IV)
12. muscle phosphorylase (Glycogen disease, type V)
13. liver phosphorylase (Glycogen disease, type VI)
14. phosphorylase kinase (Glycogen disease)
15. glycogen synthetase (Glycogen disease)
16. phosphofructokinase (Glycogen disease)
17. galactokinase (Juvenile cataracts)
18. galactose-1-phosphate uridyl transferase ("Galactosaemia")
19. fructokinase (Benign fructosuria)
20. liver aldolase (Fructose intolerance)
21. L-xylulose reductase (Congenital pentosuria)

Disorders of amino acid metabolism

22. phenylalanine hydroxylase (Phenylketonuria)
23. p-hydroxyphenylpyruvic acid oxidase (Tyrosinaemia)
24. homogentisic acid oxidase (Alkaptonuria)
25. cystathionine synthetase (Homocystinuria)
26. cystathioninase (Cystathioninuria)
27. histidase (Histidinaemia)
28. tyrosinase (Albinism)
29. arginase (Argininaemia)
30. argininosuccinase (Argininosuccinicaciduria)
31. argininosuccinic acid synthetase (Citrullinaemia)
32. ornithine transcarbamylase (Hyperammonaemia)
33. carbamylphosphate synthetase (Hyperammonaemia)
34. ketoacid (branched chain) decarboxylase (Maple syrup urine disease)
35. iodotyrosine deiodinase (Goitrous Cretinism)
36. proline oxidase (Hyperprolinaemia)
37. hydroxyproline oxidase (Hydroxyprolinaemia)
38. valine transaminase (Hypervalinaemia)
39. isovaleryl-Co.A dehydrogenase (Isovaleric acidaemia)
40. lysine-ketoglutarate reductase (Hyperlysinaemia)

Mucopolysaccharidoses and sphingolipidoses

41. glucocerebrosidase (GAUCHERS' disease)

TABLE 4—*continued*

42. arylsulphatase-A (Metachromatic leucodystrophy)
43. ceramide trihexosidase (FABRY's disease)
44. sphingomyelinase (NIEMANN-PICK disease)
45. β-galactosidase (Generalised gangliosidosis)
46. α-fucosidase (Fucosidosis)
47. β-acetylhexosaminidase (TAY-SACHS' disease)

Miscellaneous disorders

48. xanthine oxidase (Xanthinuria)
49. orotidylic pyrophosphorylase and orotidylic decarboxylase (Oroticaciduria)
50. hypoxanthine-guanine phosphoribosyl transferase (LESCH-NYHAN disease; gout)
51. serum cholinesterase (Suxamethonium apnoea)
52. methaemoglobin reductase (Methaemoglobinaemia)
53. catalase (Acatalasia)
54. "alkaline phosphatase" (Hyppophosphatasia)
55. sulphite oxidase (Neurological damage and lens dislocation)
56. pancreatic lipase (SHELDON's disease)
57. isomaltase and sucrase (Sucrose and isomaltose intolerance)
58. lactase (Lactose intolerance)
59. phytanic acid α-oxidase (REFSUM's disease)
60. NADH oxidase (Chronic granulomatous disease)
61. trypsinogen (Failure of protein digestion)
62. enterokinase (Failure of protein digestion)
63. glutathione peroxidase (Congenital haemolytic disease)
64. glutathione reductase (Congenital haemolytic disease)
65. adenosine triphosphatase (Congenital haemolytic disease)
66. lipase, "lysomal" (WOLMAN's disease)
67. lecithin: cholesterol acryltransferase (Familial serum cholesterol ester deficiency)
68. oxo-glutarate: glyoxalate carboligase (Primary hyperoxaluria)
69. D-glyceric dehydrogenase (Primary hyperoxaluria)
70. methylmalonyl-Co.A carbonyl mutase (Methylmalonic acidaemia)
71. proprionyl-Co.A carboxylase (Hyperglycinaemia)
72. uroporphyrinogen III cosynthetase (Congenital erythropoietic porphyria)
73. carnosinase (Carnosinuria)
74. acid phosphatase, "lysosomal" (Failure to thrive)

portion are removed as recognised industrial waste. Even then, the regulations governing its final disposal do not prevent abuse. The only metals being routinely monitored either in the environment or in the body are lead, chromium and mercury, although statutory clinical examinations are also carried out by the Employment Medical Adviser. Yet we now have evidence that the metabolic effects of trace metals do become overt and, in certain people, and I emphasize certain, can cause specific though probably more frequently non-specific symptoms.

Clinical experience of heavy metal effects in most hospitals has almost entirely been limited to lead in the children's department and to metal sensitivity in the skin departments. Despite the geographical location of many district general and teaching hospitals close to most of Britain's heaviest concentrations of industry, relatively little clinical evidence of industrial intoxication in the specific sense has presented. There may be two reasons for this: (1) the obvious, that little or no absorption is taking place; (2) that although absorption of metals is occurring, their effects are either non-existent, minimal or unrecognised. The first is absurd and we are left with the probability that toxic effects are minimal in a large proportion of the exposed population and do not erupt into recognisable clinical pictures. The evidence for this is scanty, and there is no reason to believe that populations differ in this respect in different industrial areas. It is probably true to say that most patients with overt symptoms in this country who have had an industrial metal poisoning have initially attended their own general practitioner, but the correct diagnosis is often arrived at late in the investigation. An index of suspicion has usually been lacking until an outbreak has alerted the medical profession. The reasons for this are not far to seek: the training of doctors in industrial medicine has never been more than a minimal part in their general training, with the shining exception of Newcastle: the level of environmental pollution within factory premises is reasonably controlled by the provisions of the Factories Acts, the factory inspector and the still too few industrial medical and hygiene services: more nebulous, the general level of personal and domestic hygiene and nutrition of today's workers in Britain may be sufficient to counter the effects of personal absorption. Finally, the genetically susceptible population may have become much smaller. Every now and again any of these conditions may alter.

Early in 1972 a small "outbreak" of lead absorption occurred in a local factory which converts scrap lead into bars by a melting process, during which the temperature of the molten lead (melting point 330°C) is raised above 500°C, sufficient to allow the vapour pressure of lead to produce a high atmospheric concentration of metallic fume. This fume then causes the deposition of lead oxide dust on the surface of the molten metal, called in the trade "dross". If this is not carefully removed by extraction and skimming, it is spread around the work area with inhalation of the dust: this is still likely to happen unless the skimmed dross is wetted and carefully stored in covered containers.

In the situation which arose, twenty-one men were found to have absorbed lead to a greater extent than the level recommended, although none of them had evidence of lead intoxication.

It cannot be emphasised too strongly that a biological screening programme, that is one which measures the effect on the human or animal body, should consider the many factors which could influence exposure, absorption and the effects on the metabolism by metals, chemicals and indeed any environmental contaminant. Such a multivariate approach is the only useful one: it is from an analysis of the several or many factors that discrimination against chance differences can be made and the relevance assessed.

Judicious programming is a difficult thing to accomplish, but time spent in preparation is invaluable. Some examples of the type of although none of them had evidence of lead 8ntoxication.

TABLE 5

The social environment	The individual	The working environment	Category of job
TYPE OF HOUSING	Age	Location of job	Manager
No. of rooms	Sex	Potential	Technician
No. of people in house	Height/Weight	toxicants	Admin.
?Source of domestic		Laboratory	Professional
water supply	Race	Foundry	etc.
Urban/Rural/Suburban	Married state	Shop Floor	
Distance to work	Smoker	Store	
Alcohol intake	"Pot" or drugs	etc.	
Dietary habits	(self or doctor		
(U.K./other)	prescribed)		
Car Driver	Selected laboratory		
"Do It Yourself" hobby	haemoglobin		
Gardener	Proteins in blood		
	?Enzyme deficiency		

14 New Industrial Techniques and their Possible Effects

1. PHYSICAL TECHNIQUES   1.1 Microwaves
                                          1.2. Laser beams
                                          1.3 Ultra-sound
2. CHEMICAL TECHNIQUES   2.1. Polymers
                                          2.2 Pesticides and herbicides
3. BIOLOGICAL TECHNIQUES   3.1. Enzymes
                                          3.2. Viruses

The increasing complexity of modern industrial methods may create a fear in our minds over the safety of workers similar to our growing concern about the potential harm of food additives and the pollution of the atmosphere. Most people are prepared to admit the possible danger of things they can see, but by no means all, as exemplified by the still heavy incidence of preventable accidents at work or in the home: invisible hazards, psychological or physical, are more difficult to keep in mind. I am going to discuss a few of the newer industrial techniques, their potential or real dangers and the protection of workers.

We can, for the sake of clearness, divide them into three categories.
1. The electro-physical
2. The chemical
3. The biological

The list is not complete but is representative of the pattern of progress and change in industrial technology.

ELECTROPHYSICAL TECHNIQUES

Microwaves. Most of us are reasonably certain of what is meant by

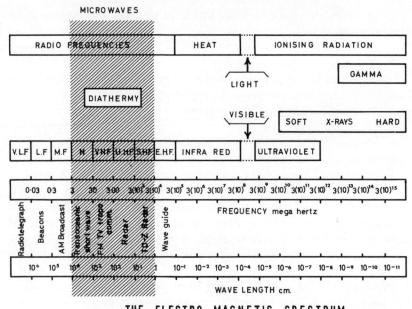

THE ELECTRO MAGNETIC SPECTRUM

Fig. 19 Electromagnetic Spectrum. The microwave band is the shaded area.

radio waves, which are a portion of the electromagnetic spectrum, much in the same way that each of the primary colours is a portion of the visual spectrum. The electromagnetic spectrum contains waves which vary from the very long radio waves to the very short radar, television and even shorter microwaves; then follow the infra-red (heating) waves, the visual spectrum, through the ultra-violet waves and on to the ionising radiation waves which include X-ray.

The effects of microwaves on animal tissues, including human, are to produce heat: in live tissues with a good blood supply this heat can be carried away and lost from the body, through the skin. In tissues with a poor or absent blood supply, such as the lens of the eye, rapid heating can occur with tissue destruction: this is the principle of cooking by microwave. The food is rapidly heated from the inside, the heat being unable to escape.

The industrial and technical uses of these microwaves may expose workers carrying out tests and maintenance on microwave quick-drying heating units used in the printing industry and other processes, microwave generators in the communications industry, microwave cooking apparatus, food sterilisation and rubber vulcanisation, to name but a few.

Short-term exposure to high intensity or long term to medium intensity can result in severe destruction of internal organs without obvious burning of the skin.

Prevention and protection are the only courses to take for those working on radar apparatus, television masts, in laboratories or in industry; three measurements should always be made:

1. Intensity of the radiation energy.
2. Duration of exposure.
3. Specific frequency or wavelength of the radiation.

Special testing equipment is available for 1 and 3.

Experimental work on animals has suggested that treatment in the event of a massive over-exposure should consist of artificial respiration, the administration of oxygen and rapid cooling of the surface of the body. Special care must be given if the abdomen has been exposed to even relatively mild doses because the hollow organs, particularly the gut, may be severely injured, may rupture and cause a rapid state of shock.

Protection of the eyes: the need to protect the eyes should not in fact arise, because no exposure above a certain specified intensity should ever be allowed. A wire screen with fine mesh will offer some protection but limits the vision of the person wearing such goggles. Avoidance coupled with foreknowledge of possible danger is the keynote. If the eyes have been exposed the individual must be referred without delay to an eye specialist with as full details as possible of the incident.

THERE ARE AS YET NO STATUTORY REGULATIONS GOVERNING THE SAFE OPERATION OF MICROWAVES

Laser beams. Laser devices often use high voltages and precautions must be taken against electric shock and explosive failure of equipment.

The definition of a laser is a system which produces a beam of parallel waves of electromagnetic energy of great intensity. The wavelengths used are from the beginning of the infra-red band to the end of the ultra-violet. The beam is very narrow, from one-twentieth to two centimetres in diameter and the energy can be delivered either intermittently (pulsed) at high power or continuously at lower power.

The use of laser beams has now broadened into the following fields:

Reasearch in industrial, government and university laboratories.
Education in schools and colleges.
Hospitals for treatment use.

Industry, machining, welding, cutting hard and soft tissue such as textiles.

Communications; along conductors or in the open.

Range-finding, satellite tracking, altitude measurement.

For the last two, being "open" across distances, great care has to be taken to protect unwary people from intercepting the beam.

Like the microwaves, laser beams will cause most damage to the eyes, this time not to the lens itself, but the lens will further concentrate the beam on to a small area of the light sensitive tissue (the retina) at the back of the eye; this tissue will be heated and rapidly destroyed, resulting in blindness at that spot. Very high energy beams will cause more severe damage to the other parts of the eye, resulting in complete blindness.

Safety in use should avoid accidents and involves restriction of unauthorised persons to access, cautionary notices, regular before-use safety checks and safety education of all people using apparatus. Ideally the beam should be enclosed. Special safety spectacles are available to give some degree of protection, but must never be relied upon for major protection.

Regular eye examination in those potentially exposed to both microwaves and laser beams should be routine, but is not as yet universal.

THERE ARE AS YET NO STATUTORY REGULATIONS GOVERNING THE SAFE OPERATION OF LASERS

Ultra-sound. The industrial uses of ultra-sound – sound waves beyond the highest frequency identified by the human ear – involve cleaning and washing processes, welding plastics, mixing liquids, drilling, and rodent control. Workers exposed have from time complained of symptoms such as fatigue, headaches, nausea and ringing in the ears. There is some evidence that these symptoms could have been due to the transmission of the ultra-sound frequency waves along a conducting system which may consist merely of a column of air contained within an enclosure, i.e. boxes stacked together.

Prevention of damage to the hearing apparatus is accomplished by enclosing the operation, but there is as yet little evidence that ultra-sound causes hearing damage or damage to the balancing mechanism of the ear. Nevertheless it is wise that precautions should be taken.

No acute effects have been reported from the industrial use of ultra-sound; the very high frequencies used in medical treatment for separation and destruction of body tissue need not be considered in this article but do emphasise the potential danger of such powerful new tools.

CHEMICAL TECHNIQUES

Polymerisation is just one example of the adaptation of laboratory chemistry to industrial production, now carried out on a rapidly increasing scale in huge petro-chemical complexes and in small factories up and down the country wherever plastics are moulded or fabricated: now they have entered the home with the use of new types of adhesives, paints and ceramics.

Polymerisation by definition means the build-up upon a basic chemical molecule of an increasing number of chemical radicals or groups, containing a variety of substances, such as nitrogen, sulphur, chlorine, etc. It is essentially the artificial synthesis of some materials which already occur in nature and of some which do not. The chemical reaction, at its simplest, involves the addition to the basic substance – the monomer – of a second chemical compound which, by the action of a catalyst, sets up a reaction to cause the growth of the monomer into a polymer. This reaction may take place with the production of gases, fumes, heat and sometimes explosive force: therefore it may require very careful engineering control to effect a safe operation. Two examples, both of which play an increasing part in our daily lives and comfort, are the formation of polyurethane foam from the basic monomers of iso-cyanates, themselves irritating and sometimes dangerous, and the epoxy-resin adhesives used in industry and the home. Both require the technique known as the "two-pot" method, which is simply the addition of one substance to another at the time of formation of the final product, polyurethane foam or epoxy-resin adhesive. The actual mixing may, however, require to be a very carefully controlled and complicated procedure.

What are the dangers? Quite recently a man in a factory was using the "two-pot" method to make polyurethane foam insulation materials to line the walls of a refrigerated truck carrier. The materials were being sprayed together from high pressure guns. The tubing of the apparatus was faulty and burst, releasing at great speed an enormous quantity of newly-formed polyurethane foam, hot and full of irritant gas which covered the operator from head to foot; his work-mates had to peel the rapidly hardening material off him before he suffocated. Nevertheless, his lungs were considerably irritated by the gases during the very short time he was encased. The epoxy-resins also are known to cause lung irritation, but more frequently skin irritation and sensitisation.

Treatment for the acute effects of these and other chemical

procedures are the standard methods of maintaining an airway, artificial respiration and treatment for chemical poisoning: the important thing is to know what happened so that a rapid appreciation of the possible effects can be made and appropriate action – of a standard nature – taken.

Pesticides and herbicides. In these days man does not live by bread alone but by the courtesy of the agricultural pesticide manufacturers, who have, over the past twenty-five years, revolutionised the production of food. At the same time we are told that these aids to agriculture have built up a pollution in water, soil and animal tissues which may eventually threaten our continued existence. Nevertheless, judicious and controlled use of these materials continues to be of inestimable value to us and our children and will not be lightly discarded.

There are many chemical types of pesticides, but we are most interested in those which can do acute harm to either the user or the consumer; I will briefly describe three of these.

The chlorinated hydrocarbons, to which group belong D.D.T., and Dieldrin, if taken internally can cause acute poisoning with effects upon the internal organs and particularly the nervous system. They are not, generally speaking, absorbed through the skin, unless exposure has been over several days; if this is the case, decontamination by thorough washing is necessary. First-aid treatment is that for acute poisoning and requires urgent expert care.

The organo-phosphorus compounds of which Malathion and Parathion are examples, poison the enzyme processes of the body, particularly those controlling the transfer of nervous stimulation from the brain and nerves to the muscle with resulting paralysis. They are poisonous if breathed as fume or dust, taken by mouth and, most important, if absorbed by the skin. Agricultural workers are at hazard unless they take care both in handling and protecting themselves during spraying operations. Many cases of acute poisoning have been reported, some fatal. Recognition is greatly helped by knowledge of what the patient was engaged in doing. Breathing may have stopped or be very shallow and the pulse may be very slow; movement generally may be paralysed. Salivation will be marked and the patient may drown in his own saliva. Desperate action is required and the quickest means must be used to get the patient to a doctor, whether outside or inside a hospital, all the while maintaining respiration and preventing saliva draining into the lungs. The doctor should be told of the possible exposure to the chemicals and will, if he confirms the diagnosis, inject Atropine in large and repeated doses. This has the effect of drying up saliva production and neutralising the paralysing action of the chemical on the enzymes of the body. A very important thing to remember is that the poison may be in the body in large quantities and, while specific treatment may be temporarily successful, unless the patient is kept under constant observation for some hours, return of paralysis may occur. Special measurements of the level of the enzymes in the blood enable the condition of the patient and the amount of treatment to be judged.

The introduction of the selective and particularly the non-selective weedkillers, notably Paraquat, has achieved some notoriety within recent years following the attempt at total lung transplantation in Britain on a boy who had accidentally drunk some Paraquat, sold commercially under the name of "Weedol". The material is a violent irritant of the body tissues, can be absorbed through the skin and is thus a very dangerous industrial and domestic poison. It causes, after absorption, severe and rapid damage particularly to the lungs, which become unable to achieve the normal exchange of gases, oxygen absorption and carbon dioxide excretion: death has been reported more frequently than recovery. Again, once ingestion is suspected, rapid transport to hospital is imperative. If splashing of the skin should have occurred before signs of poisoning, the skin must be washed thoroughly with running water, and clothing which has been contaminated must be discarded for thorough cleaning. The possibility of this type of poisoning should be constantly in the mind when a patient is known to have drunk something out of a bottle by mistake – the victims are usually young children or people who were drunk and searching for more alcohol.

BIOLOGICAL TECHNIQUES

These have been with man since he rose from off four legs and began to use his hands, a "manufacturer" in the primitive sense. We know that he has been affected by the products of animal tissue since earliest recorded history. Two recent innovations have, however, caused some concern as occupational bacterial infection itself did before means were found to control it: an example of this was "wool-sorters" pneumonia due to anthrax bacteria.

Dusts containing protein-destroying enzymes: attempts to find methods of producing brighter, whiter clothes have, within the past few years, caused the introduction into synthetic washing powders of protein-destroying enzymes, which eat away at the most resistant dirt and perform their job very effectively. However, during the earlier manufacture of these powders, quite severe effects upon the breathing of workers making them began to be noticed and it was soon found that certain people would react violently to breathing dusty air contaminated with the enzymes. Recently much stricter control of manufacturing methods has eliminated, to a great extent, the likelihood of a person developing symptoms, which are very similar to asthma. The possibility that housewives might also be affected has been a subject for some concern but so far there is no evidence of this happening. The illness has presented quite acutely with symptoms such as stuffiness of the nose, sneezing attacks, breathlessness, cough, chest pain, shivering attacks, faintness and a feeling of being unwell. Thus, if a person who works in a detergent factory develops such symptoms, he or she may have become sensitised to the enzymes, themselves derived from bacteria. It should be emphasised that this type of effect will only involve a proportion of people exposed. Treatment is confined to reassurance and calming of anxiety and the early referral for specific diagnostic testing. Avoidance of further exposure to the environment is wise until the diagnosis has been confirmed.

Virus infections associated with medical research and treatment: the history of medical research and development is marred by the tragedies of those who have died in its service. The pace of development today is accelerating: research is now an industry by nature of its size, the methods used and the quantity of products it turns out; an example being poliomyelitis virus vaccine. To prepare and grow virus, which is then inactivated by certain chemical processes to make vaccine, requires the presence of animal tissue, for it is only in animal tissue cells that virus particles will grow. These animal tissues may themselves, unknown to those handling them, contain other viruses against which there is no known protection. Such a situation developed recently when a fatal virus disease broke out in laboratory workers who handled the kidneys of vervet monkeys (*Ceropithecus aethiops*) imported from East and Central Africa. Poliomyelitis virus was to be grown in them for production of vaccine. The disease has come to be known as "green monkey disease" and is caused by the Marburg virus, after the German university town where the first outbreak occurred.

Nearer home another serious, though not necessarily fatal, virus infection has involved medical, nursing and other staff of artificial kidney units, who may have had contact with the blood of patients undergoing treatment and the blood supplied by donors to blood banks, which is used to prime the machines. This is the virus which causes serum hepatitis, a very severe liver disease, from which a number of hospital staff have died. These examples of virus infection are presented not to frighten, but to make you aware that those engaged in the Healing Industry are constantly exposed to the infections of their patients and of the materials used in preparing drugs and vaccines to heal the sick and prevent disease. Recently at my hospital, a girl worker in a commercial medical research production unit was admitted with a poisonous snake-bite sustained during the course of her daily work which was feeding snakes and extracting venom to be used in research to develop an anti-blood-clotting drug.

I hope that the examples of modern industrial practice I have given you will stimulate an interest and awareness of the techniques now being used.

In conclusion, to place our thinking in the right perspective, it must be remembered that the greatest man-made dangers to health and safety in this country are cigarette smoking, road accidents and accidents in the home. All of us have a part to play in reducing these.

15 Rehabilitation

Two Government Reports were published towards the end of 1972: the Robens Report on the Safety and Health of Workers and the Tunbridge Report on the Rehabilitation of the Sick and Injured. In each case reading them has brought a distinct feeling of *deja vu*, for in the case of the Robens Report we had the Dale Report of 1951 and with the Tunbridge Report it was the Piercy Committee of 1956. In neither instance have their recommendations been implemented to any extent. Can it be wondered that two of the largest grey areas in our health and social structure today are occupational health and rehabilitation?

An effective method of overcoming an anxious and difficult problem is "talking it out" – we seem to have been saturated recently with government reports doing just this about situations and amenities apparently necessary to our well-being but which, because of their failure to capture interest and imagination, have never made the top league. That the medical profession has failed to take up the challenge is clearly implied from paragraphs 54 and 116 of the Tunbridge Report when it says: "... However, with few exceptions, medical schools have not followed the Piercy recommendation to include rehabilitation as an integral part of undergraduate or of postgraduate study ... it is quite clear that there will be a considerable problem in finding a sufficient number of consultants to take charge of the new rehabilitation units."

In this chapter we are concerned with the return if possible of those who have been sick and injured to their former occupation, or if this is not possible that they should be retrained for a job which enables them to retain their interest in life and their standard of living.

Rehabilitation, resettlement, redeployment, reinstatement, reablement: different words, same meaning; but often different routes to the goal. In some countries they do not accept the necessity to wait for illness or accident to arise before taking steps to ensure that workers have every chance of remaining in employment, and have developed what might be described as prehabilitation. This is the withdrawal, at regular intervals, perhaps every two years at ages up to 60, from the regular employment to undergo organised mental and physical recreation together with positive health education designed to prevent the onset of degenerative disease and mental inflexibility. For industrial workers who are prepared to accept a modicum of discipline, temporary separation from families and what amounts to a considerable disturbance in their life, these schemes are both attractive and apparently worthwhile in terms of positive health and economics. They are normally carried out in places of great natural beauty and aesthetic surroundings and are best illustrated in our Western culture by the activities of the different industrial insurance schemes in Western Germany. Eastern block countries have made great use of them for many years. They may be considered effective industrial counterparts of the religious retreat and are designed for a similar purpose, a pause for refreshment and re-strengthening of the body and spirit. In this country we do not possess these facilities and neither, I suspect, do we possess the social and industrial discipline to accept them if they were offered. Yet they are not very far removed from the athletic and intellectual training camps which have become a popular and necessary prelude to successful performance, but where the motivation is clearly to attain excellence.

When a man or woman is suddenly removed from the familiar pattern of their working life through illness or injury, the impact may be delayed and cushioned by the urgent necessity for immediate treatment; recovery is later supported by the provision of the social security benefits and National Insurance payments. These have been further modified by special allowances and earnings-related payments until, in a significant proportion of cases the point has been reached, alluded to in the Tunbridge Report, where the cash payments of sick benefit, with in some cases payment of rent and rates, removes the incentive to return to work – the differential may have disappeared. I have personally spent considerable time persuading people to return to work in sheltered employment, knowing full well that while the cost of transport may be partially offset by a subsidy, yet the total "earnings" may in fact drop. It is against this background that much of the resettlement into industry has to be viewed. It is time-consuming, frustrating and often dispiriting: those involved in this work, particularly the officers of the Department of Employment and the Disablement Resettlement Officers, earn our fullest respect for the work that they cheerfully undertake. They need a missionary zeal and fortunately many of them have it.

While there has been some progress over the last forty years in the development of industrial rehabilitation programmes under what are now the Department of Employment and the National Health Service, aided by a host of voluntary organisations, industry generally has remained aloof from involving itself in what should be an important part of its social responsibility to the community. To a certain extent this can be understood, because in most circumstances the facilities to provide a reinsertion of people into their old jobs or a redeployment into new following a period of retraining are themselves expensive, putting heavy strain on smaller firms. Large organisations are better placed to do this both in the financing but, more relevant, in the staged resettlement of a worker during the reintroduction period. Once again I would remind you that the mass of this country's industrial enterprises are small firms, where there is little or no scope for redeployment. On the other hand one would have thought that the re-employment of someone who has been away sick or injured would be an urgent necessity, for in a small firm a single individual's absence can leave a large gap in the work-force. Indeed there are many small employers who are alive to this problem and do make considerable efforts to facilitate an early return, particularly by the provision of suitable transport for temporarily disabled workers. But their lines of communication are often inadequate; they don't know in what way they can help the worker and themselves. Those small firms who, through one means or another, have access to occupational medical or nursing assistance are in a better position to resolve their problems: this is one of the major benefits of belonging to a group industrial health service.

While the Tunbridge Report on Rehabilitation is mainly and rightly concerned with the deficiencies in the hopsital service, it recognises the considerable difficulties of facilitating the return of the convalescing patient back into his work. Over seventeen years ago the Piercy Committee recommended the establishment of suitable clinics in the hospital to assess a patient's fitness and progress before and after discharge. Only one-third of the hospitals in this country have followed this advice, which was essential if the difficult problems of liaison, communication and understanding of the patients' and employers' situations were to be overcome. To give you some idea of the composition, and from this the time factor involved, the following people conferring together are considered essential for assessing an individual patient's position.

Doctor responsible for patient in hospital.
Doctor (if any) in charge of rehabilitation service in hospital.
Patient's general practitioner.
Disablement resettlement officer.
Psychiatric social worker.
Medical social worker.
Psychiatrist.
Officer of the local health authority.

There is, in my opinion, one major omission, and that is an occupational health nurse or doctor who would be able to interpret the working conditions and map out a progressive return to full productivity. The dearth of such people who could afford the time and have the necessary experience entirely precludes their involvement. However, at least one large factory, alluded to in the Tunbridge Report, has for many years involved itself in this manner with the hospital rehabilitation services: Vauxhall Motors at Luton have set a pattern for others to follow; an outstanding example of what can be done for workers, the community and the shareholders!

Some years ago a colleague of mine in Lancashire set out to repair this deficiency among the small firms in his care. After some years he was forced to conclude that the time and effort of a single occupational health doctor could not be justified from an examination of the long-term results: it needs everyone involved with the patient, from the beginning of his illness to the end of his convalescence, to unite with local and central government officers and the industries themselves to sustain a successful and on-going programme.

For those of you who wish to be informed of what has been done and, more important, needs to be done, and are anxious to see that it is done, I commend to you the report of the Committee on the Rehabilitation Services for the Sick and Injured.

Lest you by now may feel despondent, that nobody cares and little is done, a brief review of some of the active programmes in different fields of medicine and industry will help you to a more balanced understanding.

As our social and medical developments have proceeded, so the demands for the maintenance of a good quality of living after illness and injury have followed. The introduction of hospitals, the motor car and hard-top roads into Africa and other developing countries has created a crisis of rehabilitation among the maimed which in some cases threatens their whole health and social programmes. We have a comparable situation in this country. Not only traffic accidents, but the techniques of modern treatment, the implants, transplants and artificial kidneys must in all conscience be followed by the rehabilitation of these unfortunate people into the community to earn their living. But for science and technology they would have been dead, and no problem. Again, as we have seen earlier (Chapter 5) the successes of the diagnosis and treatment of mental illness have led to significant reorientation of our approach towards mental illness itself but more specifically to finding productive and remunerative work for mental patients to do. Not only those who have recovered from a temporary illness but those with more serious underlying disease who remain under observation and treatment.

I believe that rehabilitation is dependent on a degree of leadership among those responsible for treatment, which is not at all commonly found, particularly now that much hospital care has become diffused into several hands. The enormous successes in returning men and women to full health and activity during the 1939–45 war were dependent upon enthusiasm and team spirit which can still be found, particularly among those who have come to command respect for their work in the neurological field in such institutes as the Stoke-Mandeville Hospital in Buckinghamshire, in the fields of clinical medicine where "Progressive Patient Care" has injected a dynamic quality into a patient's recovery not only in the application of specific treatment but in his surroundings and activity; among the doctors working with patients who have suffered heart attacks and who must be helped psychologically and physically to regain their *joie de vive* and strengthen, not coddle, their damaged hearts. Again a few industrial groups in this country have for many years accepted the responsibility for looking after their own unfortunate victims, and among these is the coal-mining industry.

It has been wisely said that when a worker is injured, not only is he damaged in body and mind but, in his own estimation, he may be damaged socially, professionally and in the regard of his own family. All the props which he needs for support are suddenly pulled away from under him. And "props" is a good expression to use if we are discussing the coal-mining industry for the miner well appreciates the value of the props he can see at his work in the pit. Miners are very often members of a close-knit, closed community, separated by a social and cultural divide from their industrial or rural neighbours. They are therefore prone to look to themselves for help and re-employment and this has in the past been a major component in their stability. But in recent years, with closures and reorganisation, fewer men have come into the industry, the age structure is narrowing towards the upper level, while modern engineering techniques have disrupted and undermined their traditional sodality. With all this is should be remembered that underground coal-mining, along with deep sea-fishing (Chapter 8)

are the most dangerous occupations we ask our workers to undertake. Both in their development of rehabilitation centres for the
injured and in the resettlement of those men whose lungs have been
permanently damaged by inhaled dust, the coal-mining industry
has beeen a good example of "do-it-yourself". This has required
much patience, not a little stubbornness, but overall the miner has
a belief in himself and his job which goes a long way to support the
needs of the industry, a major component of which is a good accident
prevention and rehabilitation service.

Perhaps it is not generally appreciated that the vast majority of
men and women who suffer acute heart attacks (coronary thrombosis, myocardial infarction) recover sufficiently to return to their
previous job. The cause of the condition is a sudden final clogging
of the main blood vessels supplying the heart muscle, which then
suffers acute insufficiency of oxygen and other nutriments and ceases
to function over a greater or lesser area with death of the muscle
tissue and its later replacement by a fibrous scar. If the area is large
or the site of the damage close to certain vital conduction paths, the
heart may suddenly stop, but oftentimes it beats on with reduced
vigour and effectiveness. With care and a little good luck, the
scarred area will shrink, the blood supply will improve if properly
stimulated and the heart continue to function for years. It is in the
growth of the blood suply that rehabilitation is of such importance:
it is no good making all sorts of plans for the future if the essential
component of recovery, the ability of the heart muscle to function
effectively in response to reasonable demands, is not provided for.
Effective rehabilitation means graduated work starting as soon as
possible which, as in all muscles, will create a response by an increase
in muscle size and, most important in this context, in the blood
supply to meet those requirements. This philosophy has governed our
thinking in this country over the past ten years. Prior to that, and
still to this day in many other countries, rest rather than graduated
and measured exercise has been the watchword. Today 80 per cent
of those patients who have had an acute heart attack return to work
within six months without having any special or prolonged rehabilitation: most will in fact be working within three months. This
contrasts with a figure of 50 per cent as found in Eastern Europe
which favours prolonged and carefully supervised convalescence.
Why this significant difference? It has been found possible to grade
severity of damage and relate this to the amount of exercise and
other special measures which may be required. But above all, as in
most illness, it is the moral component which is so important. Thus
early return to a seemingly normal existence can reduce this load of
anxiety so often provoked by over-protection when it can be shown

that this is not required. As a result of the current policy, less than 10 per cent of those in the government rehabilitation units are heart patients (see Table 1) and about 60 per cent of those who do find their way to these units are employed within three months of leaving the units.

TABLE 1

SHOWING THE PROPORTION OF SOME OF THE MORE COMMON PATIENT DISABILITY GROUPS ATTENDING THE INDUSTRIAL REHABILITATION UNITS OF BRITAIN IN ONE YEAR

Diagnostic group	Number admitted in 12 months	Total
Heart disease	998	8·4
Lung disease	1,418	11·9
Nervous disorders	1,541	12·9
Mental disease	971	8·2
Epilepsy	537	4·5
Spinal injuries	962	8·1

By physiological studies it has been found possible to relate the energy costs, and this means the demand on the heart, to the kind of work required. While they cannot for a number of reasons be used routinely on individual patients, they do serve to give a fair degree of reassurance to those who have to handle these problems of cardiac rehabilitation because they can be measured against activities which are already psychologically acceptable, for instance walking. It is important to follow these figures with a fact which is of great significance to industry and which is by no means generally appreciated. Patients who have had an acute heart attack and are once again at work have an average sickness absenteeism in every way comparable with apparently healthy men.

Doctors trained in hospitals and continuing to work there do not on the whole have the interest or zeal to supervise the recovery of their patients much beyond the hospital ward. The failure to implement the recommendation to improve the training in rehabilitation made by the Piercy Report has resulted in the present deficiencies although, as always, there can be found places of excellence sparked by enlightened leadership. Like so much of medicine today, the needs are changing, but undergraduate and immediate postgraduate training is still failing to emphasise either the modern requirements or an appreciation of the accelerated changes in

TABLE 2

ENERGY COSTS IN CALORIES PER MINUTE

Various activities and occupations

Typing	1·5	Bed-making	5·4
Watch-repairing	1·6	Carpentry	6·8
Armature winding	2·2	Beating rugs	7·0
Radio assembly	2·7	Swimming, cycling,	
Driving a car	2·8	walking	7·8
Sewing at machine	2·9	Mowing lawn by hand	7·7
Bricklaying	4·0	Felling tree	8·0
Plastering	4·1	Shovelling	8·5
Wheeling barrow 115 lb.		Planing by hand	9·1
(52 kg.) at 2·5 mp.h.	5·0	Squash	10·2
Dancing	5·2	Slag removal	11·0
Gardening	5·6	Stairs, 22 lb (10 kg) load	16·2

priorities, principally the importance of prevention, the study of the individual in his environment and his reactions to it, the after-effects of modern treatment, many of them social involving the rehabilitation of the sick and the maimed, the alcoholic, the drugged, and the aged. The statement in the Tunbridge Report that the person in charge of a hospital rehabilitation unit must be a consultant, "any consultant who comes from any discipline provided he has the necessary interest, experience and training and can devote sufficient time to the work", is at most a half-measure. It will need more than that, for the interplay between a patient's hospital illness, his general practitioner care and his reintroduction into the working community demands qualities which are not often to be found except in those working in that community, and they need not be hospital doctors. The success of full-time Rehabilitation Officers in specialised orthopaedic units serves as an example. Nevertheless, provided the medical profession adapts itself to these pressing needs and accepts the changing emphasis from traditional patterns of diagnosis and treatment, its members will still be uniquely positioned to provide the non-sectarian leadership required in such a difficult and often delicate operation as industrial rehabilitation.

Lest we forget, it is the familiar place, the familiar faces and the familiar tools which are predominant in speeding a return to full capacity. The longer a person is away from his work, whether occasioned by accident or illness, the less the chance of any return at all. Add to this the vexed question of insurance compensation and we compound the problem. Early return to work, early and interim payment of insurance or compensation can produce wonders, but where can we look for the leadership?

That signs point to the government's and profession's awareness is suggested by the establishment of the first two university Chairs of Rehabilitation in this country. They will be at Edinburgh and Southampton for the purpose of encouraging training in and development of rehabilitation of sick and disabled people. They have been endowed by the government and the National Fund for Research into Crippling Diseases in association with the Thistle Foundation respectively revealing at last a firm resolve by central government and voluntary organisations to deal with this often vexed but desperately important problem.

16 Redundancy and Retirement

"How is a nation going to keep 8½ million retirement pensioners happy in 1976? If both men and (more certainly), women are to be older longer than they were were at school, what will it take to keep them from being the most discontented political force in the country? They will be fit enough to march and could be a rival to student power." (Rt. Hon. Douglas Houghton, 1969.)

Some people might consider this fanciful, in the knowledge that discontented folk do not long retain their health, and thus the problem would be self-limiting. Add to this a reasonable assumption that work is a necessary evil for the maintenance of health in the minds of the great majority of people, particularly those who did not have the benefit of a prior educational opportunity, which might have fitted them for greater adaptability. Actuarial studies show that the possibility of a long life is no longer a pipe-dream (see Table 1), but at present it is only those up to the age of 35 who have had access to the longer compulsory education and part- and full-time higher education now freely available, who can be aware of or ready to accept the positive possibilities of leisure and avoid the frustrations of the negative ones, particularly the relative lack of

TABLE 1

STANDARDISED DEATH RATES FOR ENGLAND AND WALES PER 1,000 POPULATION AGED 65–74 (TO NEAREST ROUND NUMBER)

1851		1951		1963		1970	
Male	Female	Male	Female	Male	Female	Male	Female
64	58·5	59	37	54	28	53	28

financial independence and mobility. As Prof. Michael Hall of Southampton has recently said, "We must exorcise the acceptance of retirement as 'an eventless interregnum between work and death' ".

This confirms the increasing survival of females. It is this predominance of the male deaths which accounts for the large number of women in institutions. Any reduction in male death rate will reduce the heavy female load on geriatric medicine.

While we are witnessing a world population explosion at one extreme of life, at the other we are increasingly aware of a similar, if less dramatic explosion within our own borders due to compulsory age-retirement under existing industrial policy, redundancy in later middle life and retirement for reasons of health. Now that we can look forward to a longer period in our lives of enforced leisure than we had of enforced school work, Mr. Houghton perhaps strikes a warning note among the more joyous expectancies of life free from the responsibility of earning one's living.

The natural history of retirement is really the state of health in middle and later life and who among us bothered to consider our health in later life when we were young? This is what makes so difficult the task of propaganda against smoking and similar risks. In our advanced society, which prides itself on the care of the elderly, we have become accustomed to the inevitability of retirement with the same light attitude as we accept the inevitability of death – without a thought until it is upon us, although the insurance companies do their best to remind us! There is a general unpreparedness for retirement although the government has accepted the financial responsibility; at the present mortality rates, this probably still leaves it with a substantial advantage. When the longevity figures really begin to bite, the cost of these, both indirect and direct, will have to be reviewed and the productivity of this large fraction of the population reconsidered, perhaps in like manner to the subsidised productivity of the disabled in such organisations as Remploy, the Industrial Therapy Organisation and other "sheltered industries".

Productivity of the mind or hand can only come with experience or training, preferably both. This is now accepted as shown by the establishment of industrial training boards, and the massive re-training scheme recently announced by the government. Continuing adult education in positive health is gaining acceptance, though it is not yet widely organised; however, it is gratifying to know that some industrial training boards will now consider grants for pre-retirement training. Occupation of the mind and by the hand can be expected to reduce the load on chronic hospital beds (already up to 5 per cent for those over 65), and the weight of care in general practice,

K

for between 50 and 75 per cent of those over 70 are under treatment, mostly home visits. A mind or hand, if insufficiently stimulated, withers and the normal degeneration of later years is accelerated by inactivity. Such people allow themselves to degenerate more quickly because of inadequate income, diet and environment. This is the heart of the problem before us – physical and mental deterioration – more or less rapid, dependent upon income, occupation and general health, all of which could be anticipated and supported, to provide continued activity during what have euphemistically been called "the declining years". The rate of decline depends upon many factors, perhaps most of all on a maturity of thought towards the course and quality of natural life; for most people today over 65, it is a fairly precipitous fall.

Ageing and habit tend to accentuate personality characteristics so that neurotic tendencies, which gave people difficulty when they were younger, may give even more difficulty with advancing age. An individual's industrial sickness absence pattern during his working life is of some importance in assessing the value to himself and the community as an older worker.

Three types of older persons have been described which all of us will recognise:

1. The alert, active and creative.

2. The mentally and physically well-preserved, but who have become rigid and set in their ways and policies. They are lost if cut loose from their accustomed channels.

3. Those who show an early decay, accentuated by losses in job, relations, friends, etc.

Two aspects of the industrial environment are paramount in our understanding of the plight of many individuals. First, an ageing worker is often required to continue the same pace and quality of work as in his younger years in conditions not ideal to his declining physical capacity: and here I am quoting Mr. Jack Jones of the Transport and General Workers' Union:

"At an age, sometimes under 50, when some salaried employees are in secure jobs, with a steadily increasing income, these men find they simply cannot keep up with the pace of the modern motor plant.

"They are forced to take on the more routine, sometimes obnoxious, jobs – and it is their own mates who have decided that they should not be exploited, that they should have a reasonable place in the wages structure.

"This is true at Fords as well as many other motor companies – it is a piece of practical social justice."

Today the experienced worker in industry often has to carry quite unjustified loads of responsibility because of the current defects of manpower training and availability.

Second, the suddeness with which retirement comes to many people who have denied its inevitability is often accompanied by considerable shock, which may go some way to explain early deaths following retirement in people with apparently good health. The grief, loneliness, loss of stimuli and sense of uselessness are well known accompaniments of the early days of retirement and, unless quick substitution can be made, in susceptible people their effects can be serious: what might be described as psycho-somatic death!

From experience over the past dozen years these effects can be mitigated or delayed in a large proportion of older people. First of all the maintenance of optimal health throughout life is of paramount importance and is the target to which health screening is aimed during working life. But the changing mental and physical capacity with ageing must be matched by a modification of the work load. If this is not done two consequences arise, leading rapidly to a vicious circle. The individual becomes less and less fit for the job and continuation of the job further reduces his health. Until now, because of the non-acceptance of the fact that people may need to change their type of employment more than once in the course of their working life, thus avoiding the necessity of a change in the traditional work patterns, no studies of the problems of work capacity in relation to health on a large scale have been made. Medical and social parameters of fitness for various types of activity within the general framework of "work" are not available upon which to base an opinion in the individual case, except when some obvious major illness intervenes. A study on these lines is being planned and should make it possible to decide whether greater flexibility of employment is necessary to keep individuals at work in various occupations by indicating whether or not the job itself causes ill-health. Such flexibility would lead to greater maturity in otherwise restricted individuals and, in consequence, to a better quality of retirement.

Because of our social welfare system and the widespread company-sponsored pension schemes, the idea of eventual retirement is becoming more of an accepted fact in our social milieu, although, as I said earlier, its existence may be denied by many people for different reasons. Retirement is a state of *health* governed by a state of *mind* and can be described variously as "lazy", "working", "useful", "productive", "bored", "happy", etc., which reflects very much the temperament of the individual and his or her spouse. The acceptance of retirement is tempered by disagreement as to its timing: it is the arbitrary figures of 55, 60 or 65 which are apparently so necessary for actuarial requirements, yet so indigestible by someone who feels fit enough to carry on. It is here that the provision of pre-retirement retraining, phased withdrawal from work or change of work, the acceptance of new and, one hopes, challenging opportunities in a different field, which can lead to both acceptance of official retirement and a fresh forward outlook in the third quarter of life. It is perhaps significant that "woman's work is never done" and that women on average live longer.

Earlier I mentioned what might be called "retirement shock" and it is worth examining the factors which can bring this about. The abrupt cut-off engendered in our present system is in marked contrast to the traditional non-industrial cultures where the man or woman in late middle life gives way more or less willingly to younger members of the family, yet continues to exercise an influence in holding the "extended family" together (see Fig. 1). An apparent reduction in status is accepted, though it often appears degrading to people from modern societies to see the older people occupying what amounts to a servile position in the family. Yet they do have a niche, they are kept active and busy, they do not necessarily have to make too responsible decisions and are thus allowed to "run-down" more smoothly than their modern Western counterparts. To be sure conditions may not always be ideal and one of the problems to be found is that these old people suffer degrees of malnutrition and get reactivation of tuberculosis, so common in such communities; they become the source of continuing infection to the younger members of the family. In summary so far, I think you will see that I would prefer to substitute "rehabilitation" for "retirement" and to stage this rehabilitation by continued training and education throughout life dependent upon physical or mental capacity. The concept of paying people to do nothing during retirement must have evil effects: their non-productivity places an increasing taxation burden upon the wage-earner, and their mental and physical deterioration demands an increasing quantum of medical and institutional care to be given them, reducing that available to prevent and treat short-term illness in the younger and major productive workers. Partial subsidies to reduce older people's dependence on pensions by providing work and payment could materially reduce this demand and at the same time provide manpower for certain types of work within their capacity. This would presuppose some direction of labour and the reservation of scheduled work for certain age groups or disabled people. One factor that has already limited the voluntary activation of such a programme has been S.E.T., for payment of this tax by the employer required him, in economic terms, to obtain a worker with the highest output.

This leads us to consider the position with regard to earlier retirement for reasons of health, which presents a problem, particularly in heavier industry, when compensation for industrial injury or prescribed disease does not enter into consideration. Short-term rehabilitation programmes are available for people declared unfit for their present job and the Department of Employment and Productivity Industrial Rehabilitation Units cater for such people: their absorption back into industry after retraining is the rub. But many people retired for medical reasons do not go to the Industrial Rehabilitation Units which anyway have a relatively limited scope with a short-term target, and are virtually restricted to those who have recovered from an illness leaving them with a permanent disability. Our problem is that of the cardiacs, the respiratory cripples, the vascular accidents and those with psychiatric illness. It is satisfactory to know that the picture is changing and that Industrial Rehabilitation Units are beginning to accommodate these people.

The criteria for medical retirement differ considerably both within a single industry and certainly among different industries, dependent upon set policies, size or organisation, capacity to absorb less productive people, sickness benefit and pension plans and many other more nebulous factors. In blunt terms it is often more profitable for an employer to release or retire an unproductive worker and replace him, rather than assume the cost of retraining him, either in his own plant or by some outside organisation.

This aspect of a particular industry's or organisation's policy is fundamental to any advice we can give. Too often the doctor in industry may be requested to facilitate such a retirement when the medical grounds and certainly "the best interests of the patient" do not support such action. On the other side of the coin, the family doctor or doctor in hospital may suggest to the patient early retirement without any appreciation of the company's policy, and again this could be against the long-term "best interests of the patient". In the U.K. 44 per cent retire from ill-health and 32 per cent from compulsory retirement. Both cerebro-vascular accident and coronary disease have an incidence in retired men over 65 almost double that in men still working.

At present there is no nationally agreed system for medical retirement. Assessment by a board including doctors, personnel, welfare and resettlement officers is limited to the statutory requirements governed by the Factories Acts in relation to industrial injuries and certain prescribed diseases. There are many examples of these boards, perhaps the best known being the Pneumoconiosis Panel – resettlement training, both pre- and post-retirement has been a notable feature of the pneumoconiosis programme. But a man or woman today, not employed in an industry with this sort of programme, faces a very stressful situation over and above the sickness causing retirement. Some years ago one of England's best-known cricketers was advised that he could continue to play county cricket after recovery from a heart attack at the age of 38, but to avoid the strain of test cricket – but what were the criteria governing this advice? No more than an informed guess that "in the best interest" of the patient he should continue to play competitive cricket. Yet again another cricketer who lost an eye made his own decision in the face of obvious difficulty in reaching the required standards of efficiency. The advice given to one patient may be devastating for another with similar trouble – here the personality, resilience, insight and co-operation of the patient are all important. If the lines of communication in his industry or organisation are poor, then his "best interests" may not be served by continued employment. When an industrial medical officer is able to advise, armed with the views of the patient's general practitioner and consultant, then there is the greatest hope of a satisfactory solution. The fact remains that an unproductive worker cannot be carried for very long today and must be retired, but, one hopes, with understanding of his problems and time for preparation.

In the case of mental illness the problem has been as much one of prejudice and ignorance of this kind of illness and its outcome with good medical and social care as anything else. It is often insidious in onset and thus defies comparison with a previously recognised good state of health, it is lengthy and, despite treatment, may be restrictive in eventual work capacity: this depends principally upon the type of work, form of illness, age and follow-up care. It is probably true to say that retirement for this type of disorder mainly involves the older age groups, for young mentally-ill patients are notoriously erratic, being liable to discharge themselves and so present less of a long-term problem to their employer. But among the older patients, medical retirement may be masked by an accelerated retirement put down to more general reasons: thus the size of the problem is difficult to assess. Nevertheless, since the establishment of specialised rehabilitation centres (Roffey Park, etc.), it has become clear that unless attempts at resettlement are made the "best interests" of the patient and of the community will not be served. The recent pronouncements of the increased responsibilities of the community in relation to long-term psychiatric care have brought these problems into open discussion.

It seems unrealistic to discuss retirement, medical or on other grounds, without considering the important influence of the individual's social milieu. One can appreciate that this in no way can be expected to influence a decision, but rather the form and preparation for retirement, both vitally important if the "spark of life" is to be retained.

From the viewpoint of doctors in a hospital setting or in a group practice, they need to know the extent of the problem. How often do they become involved in such decisions? The relations and communications with the employers, the patterns of illness for which retirement is recommended, the criteria used by different doctors, the assessment of social factors – all these need to be identified. One could envisage, if such a problem was shown to exist, a combined effort involving hospital, general practice, industrial medical officer, personnel officers and managers to hammer out an acceptable local answer. It would not be an easy task; having sat on a board for a number of years, one learns the immensity of problems which face both board members and the unfortunate "boardees".

I believe there is a need for industries to group themselves into associations to study their common problems of enforced medical retirement, to develop education programmes for employers and employees and to encourage greater participation in the employment of temporary or permanently disabled people to preserve at least some of their productive capacity. A lot of employers do not yet appreciate that disabled workers do have certain advantages over able-bodied, in particular their motivation and time-keeping.

I am impressed that where possible the idea of future retirement, *for any reason*, must be placed in an individual's mind a long time before the event which only premature death can prevent. People should be educated and conditioned to cope with it. That a lot of this thinking is comparatively new may come as a surprise, but in one of the most valuable books on the subject of the psychology of industry by J. A. C. Brown, published nearly twenty years ago, the word "retirement" is not to be found on a single page!

To emphasise yet again that no opportunity should be lost to set a person thinking and doing something about his retirement, here is a quotation from a wonderful old man, Alfred Aloysius (Trader) Horn, who had few peers when it came to natural wisdom:

"There's no softness about Nature. When you're driven from the herd, it's for good. I've seen a beaten old Chief weep like a child. No wounds, mind you. But his heart is broken. Aye, he knows there's no redress in a state of Nature. No newspaper talk to prop him up again. None of this so-called diplomacy. He sees Finis written all over the sunlight – same as an old elephant."

17 Health Screening Examinations

"When they wish to improve their stocks, plant and animal breeders don't hesitate to modify the environment or control inheritance by selecting one or both parents" (McKeown).

The human biologist is more limited in his ability to effect improvement in his stock, but some form of selection has been part of the course of natural events in most human population groups since time immemorial and persists to this day. "Some mothers kill their babies, some of the new babies were sick; and sometimes it is our custom to kill weak children so that others who can work will not go hungry for food given to the weak ones." This description comes from a native of New Guinea, one of the last redoubts of primitive man but is reminiscent of the cruel exposure of infants practised by the ancient Spartans of Greece to select their manhood. Today we possess more sophisticated means of improving our stock while at the same time accepting the morality of the survival of the weakest.

The health care and medical practice of tropical countries have perforce to cope with problems, sometimes on an enormous scale, with quite inadequate means when judged by standards in developed countries, while the priorities may be very different. Thus the control of endemic and epidemic disease in whole populations takes precedence over individual treatment: to achieve this, surveys to assess the breadth and depth of the problems and the correct degree of control are needed. The whole concept of screening forms an integral part of any good health programme in the tropics: this policy was later introduced among industrial populations in developed countries on either a statutory or a voluntary basis. More recently we have seen the introduction of long-term health screening programmes among the general population so far on a research basis only, the best known being the Framingham study in Massachusetts which has been following the cardio-vascular health of the town's inhabitants for the past twenty years. In this country more restricted studies have been carried out in Bedford (diabetes), Glasgow, London and elsewhere (blood fats, blood pressure and heart disease, eye and kidney disease). For many years the mass chest X-ray programme provided a self-selected screening for several millions of people in this country. In the present context we are concerned with the health of people at their work, whatever it is, comprising just under 50 per cent of the general population.

The acceptance of voluntary health screening on any scale is comparatively recent, although there have always been people from the ancient Chinese to the modern tycoon who have been willing to spend money to preserve their health rather than wait for something to happen which can be expensive and, very often more important, time-consuming. Before moving to the practical aspects of industrial health screening it is worth looking at what has led to this recent change of emphasis from traditional curative medicine in the light of new interests and possibilities encouraging people to seek better standards and quality of living.

Personal health screening has become multi-million dollar business although its effectiveness as a true preventive measure remains open to question if not to suspicion. As one American critic put it: "The Annual Physical: Factitious Farce or Futile Fetish?" The introduction of automated laboratory analytic systems and computerised assessments of standard questionnaires followed by the impersonal delivery of relevant print-out recommendations, have certainly encouraged those who bemoan the loss of personal touch between a doctor and his patient. This point of view is put very vividly by David Vaughan the actor, whose living is dependent upon good health. "The tendency to hypochondria makes it all the more advisable for me to get a regular check-up and luckily through Equity I can go every year to something called the Metropolitan Diagnostic Institute in New York where they spend half a day testing you in almost every conceivable way. Not that such tests are not grist for the hypochondriac's mill in their way, but fortunately the results come fairly quickly – some by the end of one's visit even – so at least one is not kept waiting long in suspense. Of course the whole thing is impersonal in the extreme."

The build up of such programmes initially in North America and more recently in this country and Europe has, to be candid, arisen by the nature of their promotion reminiscent of some fear rousing insurance advertisements, and the manner in which they

have caught the imagination of an influential sector of the population. These together have created a demand particularly amongst
certain levels in business and industry. Nevertheless, the exaltations
to undergo these tests reflect the constant yet understandable
anxiety of those organisations which have invested large sums for
capital equipment in setting up the projects. The constant shadow
of economic viability, as in industry itself, is sensitively responsive to
maximum uptake which requires the willingness and enthusiasm of
what is still only a limited though influential section of the public,
to spend their money on what they believe to be effective personal
preventive medicine. This has resulted within the health care field,
of promotional programmes which have sometimes offended more
conventional tastes, earning for them in turn the implication of
being reactionaries resisting the onward march of scientific medical
progress. To be realistic, if a useful programme is to be provided then
any such batteries of expensive equipment must indeed declare a
return by operating at maximum throughput. This philosophy has
been accepted within the National Health Service itself, when
deciding upon the purchase of automated and other expensive
diagnostic and treatment equipment. Not only do such devices, used
in this way, improve the accuracy and speed of results, but by
stimulating demand they reduce costs per item; the justification for
carrying out the increased numbers of tests is another though equally
contentious issue, which should rightly be decided on clinical
grounds.

Nevertheless, there are many satisfied people who have been
through these programmes and feel they have benefited more than
from the traditional cosy chat and short examination with a doctor
of their own choice. This would have been either their own National
Health general practitioner with limited time, or a fee-paying
consultation with another general practitioner or consultant. The
latter type of examination still accounts for a sizeable proportion
of all screening examinations of healthy people done in this
country.

Perhaps the strongest and best supported criticism, in my view the
most telling, is that these programmes, whether of the "print-out"
or wholly by a doctor, are highly selective by the consumer. In some
respects this is a good thing, for those who desire an examination are
most likely to be frank and forthcoming with information and
accepting advice, being concerned about their health and seeking
reassurance. The main deficiency is that those very people who might
be in most need of advice are too apprehensive to be examined or
too ignorant to accept guidance, and miss the boat completely. This
is an analogous situation to the experience gained in cervical cytology

programmes. The only way this group of people at work can come under the microscope is through a mandatory screening programme built into their job requirements: as we shall see, we are still a long way from general agreement on this.

In my opinion screening examinations should be done primarily to sustain and encourage good health, with a secondary role of uncovering disorder or disease and applying advice and correction. These roles may sometimes need to be reversed, depending upon the criteria for examination: this is an argument for the more personal assessment by a doctor at an early stage in the examination, because he is better equipped to make the distinction. A limiting factor, however, is that not all doctors accept the role of health educator. Those working in industry or health screening organisations have learnt what a valuable contribution it can be to the maintenance of good health, whereas doctors solely trained and experienced in treating established disease may find the time and effort unrewarding and unattractive. There is, too, a real danger that seeds of anxiety may be sown: sometimes this is impossible to avoid, particularly if reassurance cannot be given emphatically. Suspicion in the mind of the examiner may be communicated to the patient. In a straight treatment situation, where the patient takes himself to the doctor with definite symptoms accompanied by unequivocal physical signs, the specific treatment can usually be applied in a confident manner effectively allaying anxiety.

Presymptomatic preventive medicine introduces new techniques of interview and explanation which can be difficult to develop, not having the support of known and determinable end results. People today are immeasurably better prepared to discuss the implications of deviations from healthy living, but they are equally ready to refute what they may consider to be specious arguments. It is only when the interviewer is able to dissect calmly, assess and reassemble the separate components of an individual's working and domestic life, relating these to nebulous aches and pains and deviations from the accepted limits of normal laboratory measurements that a convincing explanation can be given.

The logistical improbability of providing the sort of programme we have been discussing for everybody whether in commerce, industry or in the professions in the foreseeable future is patently obvious, although in small populations plans are well advanced, as for instance in Sweden. Some form of selective screening is, however, a different proposition. We now have the elements of this from birth to adolescence illustrated by the examinations of mother and child before and after birth, for such faults as congenital disorders, whether of physical, infectious or biochemical nature, for example congenital hip dislocation, rubella and phenyl-ketonuria which, if not corrected, can lead to severe mental impairment. Later the school medical service identifies children who may require special health supervision, so that by the time they leave school for work or college the responsibility can be handed on to the Employment Medical Advisory Service or the student health services.

In earlier chapters (9 and 12) I have touched upon the statutory examination requirements of the Factories and related Acts, together with programmes which have been introduced by industry itself. Despite the legal requirements for working environments which dictate reasonably obtainable non-toxic conditions of dust, gases and fumes, there has not been any widespread acceptance, official or otherwise, of the differing individual susceptibility of workers when exposed to the same concentrations of unfriendly agents. But a recent government pamphlet now recognises this. "Simple tests are now available that may be used to detect those individuals hyper-susceptible to a variety of industrial chemicals (respiratory irritants, haemolytic chemicals, organic iso-cyanates, carbon-disulfide). These tests may be used to screen out by appropriate job placement the hyper-reactive worker and thus in effect, improve the coverage of the T.L.V's." The reason why some people may react adversely to certain substances while others absorb comparatively large quantities without apparent effect have been briefly discussed in Chapter 3. This inherent potential susceptibility, possessed to a greater or lesser extent by all of us may never be given a sufficient test. On the other hand, for some people life may be made miserable by discomfort if not actual disease. A man may have to give up the job he had been trained to do: he could be a motor mechanic who has developed an oil dermititis, or a transplant surgeon who carries a specific agent in his blood which could be a danger to his patients.

The simple classification into congenital and acquired traits or idiosyncrasies is being constantly extended as new answers to old problems are discovered and new materials and environments introduced to which people become sensitised. To give a few examples:

Certain fumes, gases and dusts, as we pointed out in Chapter 11, are known to precipitate among other conditions severe acute and progressive changes in the lungs. Among common industrial materials are certain hardwood and other vegetable dusts, fungi, chemical polymers such as iso-cyanates, epoxy-resins, and styrene, and some metals or their salts: nickle, chrome, cadmium, cobalt, tungsten, platinum, beryllium, and vanadium. They may cause symptoms mimicking an acute asthmatic attack or initiate a slow process of the replacement of the delicate gas exchange tissue of the lungs by scar tissue with progressive loss of function. Breathing then becomes an effort and life a burden.

Careful questioning of someone before he starts work to rule out a history of previous lung trouble or allergy is a wise precaution where potentially sensitising materials cannot be entirely excluded from the working environment. This will not provide complete insurance because sometimes it is only after a period of exposure that sensitised people may begin to react. Here again screening tests throughout employment, as for example chest X-rays and simple lung function tests, can sometimes prevent permanent changes if the worker is removed early enough from further exposure. The degree to which this type of industrial screening test is applied in this country is limited, illustrating again one of the important omissions in the statutory or voluntary health control of workers. We are slowly moving towards a better appreciation of the economic value of such tests, the argument which carries weight in industrial boardrooms. Nevertheless there are several factors which act against an effective control of this kind. These include the high turnover of labour at risk in some industries, the absence of any organisation to advise and undertake the screening systematically, and the lack of facilities in medium-sized and small firms for the redeployment of people who might be unduly susceptible.

J.C. A 35-year-old self-employed Welsh hill farmer began to have severe attacks of shortness of breath in February 1971. He noticed he had a fever with them and felt generally unwell. They always occurred some hours after he had been forking stored hay. At first he thought that he had developed asthma as his attacks were short-lived and he felt perfectly well again after his chest had cleared. But after some months the pattern changed: his chest didn't always clear up quickly, and he developed a productive cough with occasional flecks of blood. He sought his doctor's advice and the tentative diagnosis of "farmer's lung" was made, duly supported by X-rays, lung function tests and, most specifically, by blood tests. He was advised to give up farming and take a sedentary job, for his lungs were sufficiently damaged to preclude a full recovery even if he was never exposed again. Hypersensitivity to the fungi *Thermopolyspora polyspora* and *Microspora vulgaris* had developed from breathing the dust of mouldy hay. He was able to claim benefit under the National Insurance (Industrial Injuries) Act 1964 because "farmer's lung" is a Prescribed Disease (see Chapter 9). A recent change in the Act allowed his claim; previously benefit was not available to those who had been self-employed; a much criticised omission.

Screening lung function and blood tests are now available to support a specific diagnosis of "farmer's lung" and should constitute a routine diagnostic procedure in all people with suggestive symptoms who may have been exposed to mouldy vegetable material dust. Early removal from exposure results in complete recovery and these people should never again be knowingly exposed at their work. It has not yet been possible to apply blood tests, on a screening basis, to farmers. In the meantime the need may actually disappear as hay storage methods are improved sufficiently to forestall the development of these thermophilic or heat-dependent fungi. This distressing condition may soon be of historical interest only; it has been recognised for over two hundred years although its specific nature, the development of hypersensitivity to specific fungi, remained undiscovered until 1963.

J.W. A 40-year-old English carpenter first became ill in March 1970 when he developed a cough with wheezing, felt generally unwell and had to leave his work. Just before his illness he had been employed with another man, a painter who remained well, in cleaning a flue in a platinum metal refinery, but his usual work was to make and repair wooden jigs or moulds for the refining process. The ones he repaired were often contaminated with platinum salts; in the process of repair he would sand them down, creating dust. His current symptoms took a week to settle down. On his return to work he was given a specific platinum skin test and reacted strongly positive. He recalled one previous though much milder attack some months before, which didn't keep him away from work. He had been in his present job for four and a half years, and had been a carpenter for fourteen years previous to that, never with any symptoms suggesting he could have developed a wood dust sensitivity. He was a moderate smoker, twenty cigarettes daily; there was no family history of allergy. However, he did recall that for the past year or so whenever he was near bins of refinery residue being emptied, he would get a tightening of the chest followed by an irritating cough the same night. He has avoided exposure to platinum salts and has remained well since. It is now accepted that in the rare metal refining industry those with a history of allergy (not present in this patient) are more at risk: unfortunately, skin tests cannot be used for screening because they themselves may create a sensitivity where none had existed before, but they can be used to support a clinical diagnosis.

The third case illustrates the kind of problem which immigrants from countries where once malaria was heavily endemic may experience. In a proportion of the inhabitants of these countries certain bio-chemical mechanisms activated by enzymes inside the red blood cells have become modified because of selective deficiency of enzyme which reduces the chance of severe malarial infection. However, as a consequence, in the presence of other kinds of insult particularly chemical, from either pharmaceutical or industrial processes, the reduced amount of enzyme may be unable to cope with its normal activities leading to a break-up of the red blood cell and rupture of its membrane, a situation known as haemolysis; it can be fatal but is usually a self-limited condition following removal from exposure. One of the enzymes affected in this way is Glucose 6 phosphate Dehydrogenase (G6PD).

M.A. A 24-year Iraqi Arab was employed in a small industrial store receiving chemicals and redistributing them in smaller quantities. He had worked there for six months until one day he felt unwell with severe weakness and nausea: he was quite unable to do his job of tapping drums of a chemical he had not been exposed to before, hydroquinone, and filling small containers. He was found to be jaundiced and very anaemic; his urine was dark brown. A diagnosis of acute haemolytic anaemia due to a deficiency of G6PD enzyme in his red blood cells was made. Fortunately he proceeded to a full recovery without further complications. He was advised to change his job and was given a list of drugs and chemicals which he should avoid; this was necessarily incomplete as it is constantly being added to. Enquiry did produce the information that as a child, after eating the common broad bean (*Vicea fava*) in Iraq, he used to suffer attacks of weakness: they were undoubtedly of a similar nature to his recent attack. The broad bean is a well-known trigger agent in susceptible people. This unfortunate incident, arising in someone who was completely unaware of any abnormality, has been increasingly reported in recent years. In the United States it is found among the industrial Negro population. It is possible to screen such individuals by a simple blood test which is now done in the United States and in some more industrialised African and Middle Eastern countries. It occurs as a more severe condition in people of Semitic origin, both Arabs and Jews, than in Negroes. The fact that so far in this country it has not yet presented a problem is perhaps related more to chance and the relatively mild, possibly unrecognised, reaction in people of African origin than to any studied plan of prevention or avoidance. If at any time a large influx of Middle Eastern workers took place the situation could change.

The systematic examination or screening of the bio-chemical and immunological (defence against foreign matter particularly infectious agents) profiles of the many thousands of workers in industry exposed to even the known potential hazards is still a long way in the future, but as has been shown, relatively simple enquiry of personal history can often reveal sufficient information for a judgement to be made. Sometimes only the empirical test will provide the answer, and this may be acceptable provided it is done with due care and attention, avoiding unnecessary over-exposure. Too many tragedies have occurred before this was realised, so distressingly illustrated following the exposure of women workers to beryllium in the early days of fluorescent tube manufacture twenty-five years ago. A similar risk is being perpetuated by continued exposure during manufacture and handling of that useful but ubiquitous material, asbestos.

Perhaps the outstanding advantage which industrial health screening possesses is that it can make use of people who are not doctors to carry out a great deal of the basic information collection, a job which, when we were discussing the personal health programme, is often now being delegated to computers. But paramedical workers, to use a descriptive and widely inclusive term, can by the knowledge they possess of industrial and other occupational environments make a more accurate assessment and combine this with simultaneous health education. Industrial health programmes have been pioneers in the introduction and use of these people, and perhaps only reluctantly and for differing reasons have other branches of preventive health care and particularly hospital and general practice begun to train and use them. The great problem of our age, social pathology, is presenting just such a challenge, requiring both professional and non-professional training of social workers to work alongside their Health Service colleagues.

The basic elements of health education which can be beamed to people at the time of screening are, with equal emphasis, diet and nutrition, weight and obesity, regular exercise, smoking and alcohol, rest and relaxation, and personal hygiene. The history of industrial medicine has taught us that it is the additive and potentiating factors allied to a specific toxic material which can make the difference between health and disease. Many of these factors can be controlled and eliminated by the individual himself. As we have seen earlier (Chapter 11), smoking in particular has pushed many people beyond the limit of the health enjoyed by their non-smoking fellows working in the same environment.

18 The Role of Occupational Health Services in Economic Development

In retrospect, the appalling load of sub-optimal and frank ill-health among the rural and later industrial population of Britain 150 years ago was directly due to the crude exploitation of the worker and his family without thought of the effect that the working conditions had upon their health and well-being, let alone productivity. The very absence, with but few exceptions, of work-based medical services, such as for instance existed in the armed forces, could have been largely responsible for the failure to improve conditions, though it must be admitted that environmental sanitation even in the services still left much to be desired as Florence Nightingale, the critics' chief spokesman, made quite clear.

Much of the failure to take account of known factors was transported overseas into new development areas of plantation, mining and later manufacture: some of these led initially to devastating changes in the long established though always precarious balance of "health". Much the same situation still exists in many places today, but improved nutritional state and housing have softened the impact.

The argument smoulders on between employers, unions and government on the one hand and not nearly enough of the health workers on the other, that the failure to provide an overall occupational health cover in this country is at least partly responsible for the massive sickness absence figures, despite the provision of a National Health Service. The latter has had, until very recently, little interest or responsibility even for the occupational health of its own working staff.

The factors which contribute to the absenting of a worker through "sickness" are several and varied, being beyond our present consideration, but there is no doubt that from the experience gained where some of these can be controlled, a very real benefit can arise affecting not only the worker but his family, community and the commonwealth – this should equate with ordered and balanced economic growth. But any attempts to facilitate the workers' adaptation and well-being should today be carried out without the element of overt paternalism, which is no longer acceptable although in different times and places it was able to provide the template for the growth of a whole country's health services.

The compassion for human suffering is among the most precious of our cultural possessions; it has been a cornerstone in the teaching of all the ancient religions and at least one of the new ones. The traditional approach to the relief of suffering is still, and rightly so, based upon the personal care by one individual for another, but the past hundred years have shown the contribution which can be made to the often remote and necessarily impersonal care by disciplines within medicine itself and, more recently, beyond its fringe.

If I were asked what was the one factor which has made the greatest impact for good or evil on human well-being I would answer, almost unhesitatingly, "communications". Communication in all its forms has steadily narrowed the gap between ignorance, poverty and human well-being, although at times as Ronald Hope has pointed out, it has "spread man's ignorance at terrifying speed".

Industry in the past has been foremost in opening up the pathways into new development areas and providing the communications ultimately to the benefit of everyone, although it should be remembered that when the age-old tribal and cultural patterns have become disrupted and susceptibility to exotic infection has crippled a community, the benefits may not at once be appreciated! It is terribly necessary to anticipate these possibilities and provide suitable substitutes and protection – the social African tribal dancing in the Johannesburg gold-mines is an excellent example. Any development, healthwise or whatever, should be accompanied by a wide-ranging consideration of the issues and potential ill-effects – these have been too much a feature of uncontrolled industrial growth. The recent development of medical geography can contribute fruitfully to this planning; it is uniquely positioned to do so by its cross-disciplinary approach but it is necessary that it should engage the interest and respect of those who, in their separate fields, have already made significant contributions.

Industrial development influences and initiates changes within a country in many ways: three in particular are relevant to our discussion:

1. *The effect upon the topography*
   Changes can arise out of the industrial process itself, such as quarrying and mining which give rise to slag heaps and dumps: the creation of reservoirs, borrow-pits, canals: the denuding of flora by pollution. The provision of roads, railways aerial ropeways and power lines, secondary effects by a predatory population causing deforestation, erosion and shanty-towns. The ecology becomes disturbed sufficiently to allow the growth of influences harmful to man. On the other hand industry may recreate aesthetic and functional features which are a marked improvement on what existed previously.

2. *The effect upon an indigenous population*
   Urbanisation versus pseudo-urbanisation.
   In-migration and immigration.
   Diseases of aggregations → new disease patterns →
   → Transference of established susceptibilities in immigrants.
   Food shortages: hoarding: nutritional diseases.
   Increase in fertility rates → nutritional diseases such as Kwashiorkor
   Disruption of established mores → crime.
   Emergence of new social groupings
   ↓
   dualisms, racial or national segregation.

3. *The effect upon the economy*
   Balanced versus unbalanced.
   Too rapid reduction of reserves, without planned replacement (forestry, plantations, agriculture and fishing).
   Reinvestment locally of profits, secondary industry.
   Consumer goods imports versus locally produced.
   Technical assistance $\begin{cases} \text{self-help.} \\ \text{international agencies.} \end{cases}$

All of these necessarily are concerned with industry's relations with government, its own workers and help from the right quarter if there is to be a smooth transition to a developed economy. The ornanisational structure of a modern industrial enterprise at the start of operations will have a different pattern and emphasis from that of its predecessors either through its own wishes or from government pressure; this sometimes requires considerable organised environmental development before production is allowed to start. This is not to denigrate the paternalistic health and welfare organisation which have arisen over the past century in many countries, but today people wish to choose for themselves and express themselves more forcibly in the character of the changes which will take place.

The economic development of a country is closely related to the capacity of its people to adjust to change and to rise to meet the demands which industrial development imposes. Exploration, development, consolidation and production are the sequences of economic growth.

At each stage the capacity of the developers to mould and fashion industry, whether agricultural or manufacturing, will have depended upon their own quality of survival and their ability to create the necessary environment for the survival of those who provide the essential manpower. Our minds may turn to the lack of appreciation of these needs during the period when slave labour, transported from West Africa for the great plantation developments in the Americas, was freely available and apparently expendable. For the European peoples, however, the labour needed to develop their own countries was not expendable to the same extent, although initially the drift from country to town obscured the fact that the natural population growth only just allowed for replacement: without immigration the high infant mortality matched and potentiated the effects of the low adult survival rates. Despite modern cynical views the archives tell us much of the efforts that were made on man's behalf, in the context of the times, to recognise and improve the often appalling conditions in which men, women and children earned their living.

The advent of modern scientific medicine cannot alone have been responsible for the demographic changes which had already begun to accelerate in Britain and to a lesser extent in Western Europe by the mid-eighteenth and early nineteenth centuries: the doubling of the population of Britain from seven to fourteen million during the seventy years from 1760 took place at a time when the only specific medicines were mercury for syphilis and quinine for malaria! Even so the actual causes of these diseases were not then known. The recognition by employers of labour of the need to house, clothe and feed their workers, at least to a minimal standard to achieve any performance at all, was in part the reason for the growth in population. Slow improvement in the infant and child-hood survival figures was followed by an increase in adult survival rates: in retrospect a revolutionary change was achieved in the numbers and perhaps more significantly the distribution of the population in industrial Britain. These sociological advances, pitiful by our standards today, caused, in those drawn to the cities and towns, a significant increase in their family growth and fertility rates, which soon led to the vast overcrowding and degenerate conditions so sympathetically illustrated by Dickens, Trollope, Reade and other novelists. Yet in the beginning, the new "back to backs" were a real improvement on the rural hovels from which many of these people came. But the coming of scientific medicine in the mid-nineteenth century did have its effect on the infectious disease figures; they began to fall, due perhaps more to the universal recognition of their infectiousness than to any specific medical treatment. This coincided with the period when the nature of much disease was being actively investigated and classified by two new disciplines, epidemiology and pathology.

The traditional picture of the native inhabitant of the tropics sitting listlessly under his palm tree is fast becoming an anachronism. Early military and merchant venturers from temperate Western countries regarded the native of the tropics as lazy and idle and not to be relied upon if work, in the Western sense, had to be done. Apart from the instinctive wisdom possessed by inhabitants of hot countries that it was wise to keep out of the sun and conserve energy for the cooler hours of evening or early morning, most of these people were infested by parasites, competing with the body tissue for the scanty nutriment the host was able to obtain. With respect to the many forms of indigenous therapeutic medicine, no impact upon this continuous cycle of sub-optimal health was made until the causes were recognised and preventive measures undertaken: with treatment alone, the cycle could not be broken, as exemplified by the continuing problem of schistosomiasis throughout the world today.

The partnership of enlightened self-interest extending to humanitarian health services for the community, with the commercial and industrial benefits of opening up routes to trade and prosperity, may be reviewed in the light of the long-term economic and demographic effects of the medical services of the East India Company in the eighteenth/nineteenth centuries, the survival of the rubber plantations in Malaya, the mining of gold 10,000 feet underground, again in India, and the development of the oil state of Kuwait. All of these helped to open the routes to trade, industry and agricultural development: each of them had natural and man-made environmental problems of the greatest magnitude with which to cope. Without their medical services nearly all these great projects would have foundered and the world would have been the poorer in the quality of life for millions of people.

The English East India Company was clearly a pioneer both at home and abroad in industrial medicine as practiced today; one of its own surgeons said of it nearly 150 years ago: ". . . I think employees . . . enjoy advantages in the preservation of health beyond any other body of men and therefore, as a body, likely to be more healthy than the rest of society generally." Such an enlightened appreciation by an employer of the value of a man's health and the means taken both to preserve it and support him financially and medically if and when he was sick was unusual, and makes surprising reading from a period when men and women were being transported for their lifetime as punishment for petty theft!

The remote outposts of the East India Company within the Indian sub-continent and beyond, particularly in the Persian Gulf and the East Indies, required it, from the earliest days, to provide a preventive quarantine service against infectious disease, particularly cholera and smallpox, together with a treatment service for its servants, military and civil, expatriate and native. The pathetic legends upon the gravestones scattered throughout the sub-continent demonstrate the very real occupational hazard of life in India in those days. But many were able to survive and give years of valuable service: such a one was Dr. William Hamilton in the early eighteenth century. By his work and devotion, he created an atmosphere of mutual respect and trust which opened the doors to trade and industry for his countrymen and helped remove the natural suspicion of the native inhabitants. Another was Dr. Gabriel Boughton, who by his services to the Emperor Shah Jehan at Agra and later to his son Sha Shuja, Viceroy of Bengal, obtained a "firman" or grant which facilitated the entry of the East India Company into Bengal, thus allowing the first trading factory to be established on the Hooghly River as early as 1640.

The Company provided its ships and factories with doctors or surgeons and their assistants, men of sometimes exceptional calibre and staying power: the records show that several of them remained at work in India for more than forty years during the seventeenth and eighteenth centuries. Only the strongest in character and body could have survived: little is to be read of their daily mundane activities from the official reports and letters, yet between the lines the inference is clear. The profession of medicine and surgery was an honourable one, which was pursued with honesty and zeal according to their abilities and opportunities by far the majority of medical men who served the Company in its various fields. The demands for their services by princes and kings were frequent, and through such opportunities they were able to procure peculiar advantages for their employer. But of greater significance yet was their service to the people of India. "You are right in supposing that I have expressed an opinion that the peaceful and civilising influence of the work done in the dispensaries (and by regimental surgeons on the frontiers of India) has been in political importance equivalent to the presence of some thousands of bayonets. I have held this opinion, because no amount of military coercion or of purity of admission could have exercised the same pacifying effect on the heart of the nations than had been produced by the sympathetic care and successful treatment of diseases, many of which had been previously incurable. . . . The great question to be solved in the future is that of how to bridge over the chasm which separates the ruler from the ruled. The means of accomplishing this end may be mainly looked for in the sympathy to be created between the races; and I think the medical profession will always have it in their power to give most important aid towards the attainment of this object." Thus wrote the Commander-in-Chief in India in 1887.

Perhaps the greatest memorial which the Indian Medical Service, the successor of John Company's doctors, left in 1947 was the system of medical education throughout India, with over 50,000 Indian doctors trained in Western medicine at the time of partition. It is ironic that industrial Britain in 1973 has come to depend upon the later fruits of that great medical education programme, to provide just over a third of the doctors it needs for its own health services!

The work of Malcolm Watson in Malaya and Gorgas in Panama at the turn of the nineteenth century foreshadowed the integration of epidemiological, topographical and engineering techniques, essential for the successful control of insect-borne disease. They have remained models to this day, though the awareness that physical and mental disease may result from the alteration of the topography by insufficiently or badly planned engineering still eludes the thoughts of some who are responsible for development. Watson's report of his work, originally published by the Liverpool School of Tropical Medicine in 1911, was very soon sold out, showing that the time was propitious when national and local governments and industrial developers were ready to accept that money spent on prevention of disease could bear tangible results within a foreseeable time, whether those results were in the relief of human misery or the improvement of production figures. Sir Ronald Ross, the discoverer of the malarial parasite cycle in the mosquito and its warm-blooded host, wrote in the foreword to Watson's report: "The time is one of change and advancement in our ideas and colonial development. We are passing away from the older period of incessant wars and of great military and civil dictatorships into one of more minute and scientific administration in which the question is always held before us: What can be done for increasing the prosperity of the people? Sanitation is almost the first word in the answer. Prosperity is impossible in the face of widespread disease." How wrong he was about war, the instrument of vainglorious corporals and kings, but how right about sanitation, the new understanding of the nature of disease which, paradoxically, has enabled wars to be fought to a more bitter and bloody end. Now, sixty years on, we are acutely aware that sanitation and the preservation of health are not by themselves the answer, for they have combined to present us with a population explosion which threatens to create a greater unease of the mind than disease has of the body.

The work in Malaya had to start from scratch: the study of the mosquito vector, its identity, habits, breeding places, the survey and mapping of water sites, the ditches, swamps, ponds, lakes, borrow-pits, rivers, canals, irrigation channels and, where relevant, lagoons and estuaries into the sea. Watson's report is a fascinating saga of detection with many maps and photographs. He defined the population movements caused by malaria hyperendemicity which had led to the abandonment of houses and villages. He investigated the nature and effects of soil, water and vegetation in their relation to adult mosquito habits and larval breeding, and made proposals for effective drainage on a permanent scale. The work was soon extended to the newly developed area of Port Swettenham which was to serve the state of Selangor, for as soon as the port opened in 1901 epidemic malaria broke out and severe restrictions on its capacity rapidly followed. Within six weeks of the adoption of drainage and mosquito control "the work of the Port was proceeding without great difficulty".

It is worth emphasising that what was relevant to malaria and protozoal diseases yesterday is just as relevant to virus diseases today. With the identification of sylvatic foci and the transfer of mammalian infection to humans the lesson is there, whether it is yellow fever in Trinidad, "Russian" (Powassan virus) spring–summer fever in Canada, Kyasanur virus in South India or acute haemorrhagic fever in Eastern and South-east Asia.

Watson showed himself to have more than medical strings to his bow. "It is an interesting speculation how far malaria has increased in certain parts of Italy from the slow interference of drainage by geological processes. We know that the delta of the Po is gradually extending, and that during the past two hundred years the annual increase has been at the rate of 55 feet per annum. It may be, too, that slight elevations of the sea bed have also interfered with the flow of the rivers in parts of Italy, and so produced or increased malaria. We know changes have occurred in the level of the lands around the Mediterranean during the Pliocene and recent geological periods, and subject as it still is to considerable volcanic influences, it is not impossible that a hypogenic factor has caused once prosperous places to become desolated by malaria." The relevance of these remarks to the fossil estuary (Kuwait Bay) of the Wadi Batin emptying into the Persian Gulf may be significant in the disappearance of malaria from the north-eastern sector of Arabia, which I will be discussing shortly.

I believe the lesson from Malcolm Watson's work seventy years ago has not yet been learnt by some of the newly emerging countries who, as soon as they can find the money, build hospital palaces which are rapidly filled. Not only do they fail to tackle the causes of disease at their root source, but the restricted health budget is soon drained away to maintain these often unsuitable emblems of prestige, leaving little for the important fields of health education and engineering.

Most people are aware of the economic significance of the South African gold-mines, but my story will be of those in South India, which at the time of my own experience, were then the deepest underground mines in the world, reaching to a depth of 10,000 feet below the surface.

Gold in India has for many years fetched a higher price than that on the official world market. As a result, the mining of gold at Kolar in South India, which may have been undertaken since antiquity, until very recently remained a profitable industry: by the middle of this century the taxes payable to the Mysore Government had contributed in large measure to the state's economic prosperity and industrialisation, earning for it the title of "The Model State": at the time I knew it, it had just come under the control of the Central Government, with the independence of India. The four mines employed 23,000 persons, 14,000 of them underground, and supported a population of more than 125,000 people. By mid-century a depth of 10,000 feet had been reached by elliptical shafts 20 feet in diameter: at this depth the rock temperature approaches $150°F (66°C)$.

As a result of the mining methods characteristic of narrow lodes (thickness of gold-bearing quartz rock) the world over, with increasing depth mined, "rock-bursts" due to the enormous pressure resulting from the artificial faults created, are a serious problem and have led to major accidents. It will be appreciated that the safety and health of miners was a serious consideration with the increasing depth of operations, and an extensive education programme was developed.

On the Kolar Gold Field two problems arose: first the efficiency and acclimatisation of men working in high temperatures and humidity; and second, the effects of these conditions, together with dust, upon the respiratory system, predisposing it to both acute and chronic lung disease.

The South Indian miner, of Dravidian stock, is not imbued with any special characteristics which help him in adapting preferentially, although at the time he was being studied his average height, weight, surface area and diet were probably adequate for withstanding extremes and acclimatising to high underground temperatures. The evidence showed that these men were able to work efficiently at temperatures and conditions of cooling which were unfavourable to European miners in Europe. It emphasised that the key to efficiency was ventilation, but here again efficiency fell off if cooling was too effective.

To a visitor to Mysore today the significance of efficient production of gold and the health of the miner at Kolar may not be apparent. Yet the extensive industrialisation which has taken place is in no small measure a result of these earlier efforts to create acceptable working conditions for underground gold miners.

Since the discovery of natural petroleum it has become necessary for people to lead active lives in climates which had, until then, been considered virtually impossible.

Kuwait is a small state with only recently defined boundaries. It covers an area of 16,000 sq. km. between 28° and 30° north of the Equator and between 46° and 48° east of the Greenwich meridian. Bounded to the north by Iraq, and to the west and south by the al-Hasa province of Saudi Arabia, it consists of a small triangle of land centred on the Bay of Kuwait, a fossil estuary of the great Wadi Batin. Kuwait City in summer is among the hottest capitals in the world, while in winter, temperature minima approaching freezing point. Equally extreme is the rainfall which, as long as detailed records have been kept (since 1955), has never exceeded 200 mm. annually. In several very dry years less than 30 mm. has been recorded.

Kuwait greatly lacks manufacturing industry either on the bazaar level or as an organised factory system: only recently, with the sizeable resources of cheap power and chemical feedstock, has some attempt been made to combine these elements into a chemical industry.

Early in the development of modern Kuwait it became obvious that an understanding of survival at high environmental temperatures was mandatory if exploration for oil and further development of production and sea transport was to take place. For the Kuwait Oil Company the problems were twofold: hot humid atmosphere affecting port workers and tanker crews, and very hot but dry desert conditions during five summer months. A concerted approach by experiment and education, enlisting the help of the Liverpool School of Tropical Medicine, produced a significant improvement both in the morbidity from heat illness in the company workers, many of them expatriates, and among tanker ships' crews.

The factors which contribute to the escalation of the failure of the body to resist elevation of the body temperature do not arise from any one source and even yet they have not fully explained this very serious condition. In 1947 in the Persian Gulf, with the huge increase in the number of tanker crews and a concomitant heat-stroke morbidity and mortality, there was an urgent need to apply such principles as were known and reduce what was fast becoming a serious load upon the limited medical facilities in Kuwait. Early treatment and effective educational measures among the crews and tanker companies over the next few years reduced the incidence of the condition among this special population to a trickle. Coincidental with the satisfactory waning of heat-stroke in tanker crews arose a worrying incidence among the new immigrant population on land, particularly in the rapidly expanding urban areas of Kuwait, where living conditions, the absence of air-conditioning and heat insulation, led to sometimes unbearable discomfort at the height of summer. The government hospitals were receiving over one hundred cases of heat-stroke a year at this time and it was not until 1965 that the figure was brought down below this number.

Today Kuwait can boast of being as healthy a country as one could hope for, given the gruelling climate. Its problems are no longer those of physical health and disease, but rather the social and political questions which clamour to be answered, racial integration and desegregation, political representation, a widening of the income structure, opportunities for productive industry, establishment of trade unions and the dissipation of the fear of absorption by its neighbours.

This study has embraced a period of 350 years during which man has developed world-wide communications, which have allowed favoured nations a participation in the growing economic wealth of six of the seven continents. To a varying extent the development of this wealth has been achieved as a result of the control of endemic and epidemic infectious disease and the development of methods enabling man to live and work effectively in adverse climates, tropical and sub-arctic. We are on the threshold of the exploitation of the seventh continent, the Antarctic, and the ring of almost completely ice-covered continental shelf which constitutes the Arctic Ocean and its islands. But to introduce an unhappy topical note, the *Daily Telegraph* of 29th November 1971 reported the threatened closure of the Australian Antarctic bases due to failure to recruit medical staff. Sir Vyvyan Fuchs confirmed that this is a potential danger with the British Falkland Isles survey. Perhaps more than anything else this emphasises the enormity of the problems besetting people exploring and later developing new territories: while the exploration of both polar regions began no later than European penetration of the tropics, the physical conditions have been the bar to progress. Nevertheless, the requirements on which I have based my theme, the association and integration of medicine, geography and engineering in the widest sense, are nowhere more clearly illustrated than in the history of polar exploration and its sequelae, the ability of man to live and work in an utterly unfriendly cold climate. One day we will see whole communities living in artificial environments as their predecessors of today are learning to do. The exploration and development of the sea-bed will be another fascinating saga.

The prevention of natural disease, other than the ultimate and inevitable degeneration of the organism, should be the aim of all who work in the medical field; there is now sufficient evidence that this is possible in the foreseeable future. Enormous strides have already been made, sadly it must be admitted, only to be matched by the emergence of man-made illness and accident. Prevention can only come about by the harnessing of all available resources as I have briefly illustrated. In reviewing these – and there are many other examples of industrial development – one is perhaps made aware that in contrast to other fields of medical and health care, as for instance in the universities, medical schools, great hospitals and public health services, there has been a relative paucity of research and observational material, deriving from the "shop-floor" of industrial medicine, particularly of a nature that could be appreciated and relevant to conditions which have already arisen or might do so in the future in other areas of the world. There has been little integration of philosophy, planning, research or development; what has come forth has come haphazardly. In particular the great opportunity for medical teaching organisations and overseas industries to work together has largely been missed by this country, although I have illustrated one of the rare examples in Kuwait; the work of the Ross Institute in India and Africa is well known. Co-ordination of industrial medical and health work could provide the necessary knowledge of how to avoid the pitfalls and accommodate the changes which are already with us in the accelerating development of agriculture and industry. In developing countries the governments concerned are very sensitive as to who is achieving the recognition and profits from such development and have applied the principle of nationalisation to the extent that many of the opportunities for workers from this and other developed countries of practical experience, research and evaluation no longer exist over a useful period of time.

The value of a cross-cultural approach cannot be overemphasised, but as yet there is little preparation required for this either in under-graduate or postgraduate education in this country. The absence of a career structure for the field worker in overseas industrial medical and social development hampers recruitment and more certainly reduces the benefit that both the home and overseas countries can reap from the lessons of their experience.

19 Conclusion

I would ask you to consider this chapter in its logical sense as well as a valediction, because in effect I have presented you with a series of propositions based on personal experience. Before reading this book you may have been unaware how much of this thinking now engages the attention of doctors and nurses working close to industry. They need the help of others in the industrial and educational fields who are also convinced that this philosophy is sound. I hope that you will be induced to apply at least some of the suggestions which I have made wherever and however you earn your living. Working comfort and peace of mind are the major paths by which men and women can follow a fruitful existence. This old phrase lends itself to the simple but not easily realisable goal in contrast to what many are still saying: "We count our existence an offence."

No amount of medical science, by itself, will do away with the punishing sickness absence figures we endure as a nation. The care of one man for another, whether by advice or restraint or by active measures, is basic in most of us if we are allowed to follow our own feelings and, most important, make our own judgement. But today, beset as we are with pressures upon our time, personal security and safety and the lightening of responsibility of charity and kindliness by the replacement of an impersonal and omnipresent state machine, many people elect to "pass by on the other side of the road" carrying with them a false righteousness in the feeling that whatever could happen or has happened is none of their business. The whole relevance of sickness absence to actual illness has been shelved. Successive governments have themselves been guilty when they have consistently stated that the National Health Service provides sufficient cover to prevent and treat the disorders which arise during work, denying the need for more informed and available services.

At this time in our existence, when modern treatment has freed so many people from the mental hospitals and prevented others from entering them, when liberal, moral and social consciences have progressively persuaded the courts to rehabilitate rather than incarcerate wrong-doers, it has become everyone's responsibility, despite his disinclination, to accept the involvement which these changes demand. In the industrial context this may have special significance: all the greater urgency, then, that all sections of industry should demand optimum conditions rather than continue to rely on the often unsatisfactory statutory minimum. Great opportunities exist to use the reorganisation of health services now being undertaken to integrate the preventive and curative care of the health of people at work: there is little sign of them being grasped.

In the industrial field also the opportunities exist although the effort must come from the top and link up with the desires and co-operation of all levels. To do this, rather than rely upon legal persuasion and enforcement, industry should see how it can benefit and be benefited by the whole community of which it should be an integral part. One of the most enlightened and encouraging developments today is the responsibility now accepted by some large industrial organisations in seconding its staff to take part in the social services of the local community, something that had almost disappeared with the Industrial Revolution. That this spark has been kept alive is perhaps piquantly illustrated by the following dedication in a handbook given to new employees of a small chemical and plastics firm in this country which competes successfully with the giants.

"To Tom, Dick, and Harry, not forgetting Harriet and all who daily tread the path of labour. The Directors and Staff present this, their Charter of Goodwill and High Endeavour, for it is their happy intention to be on the best of terms with everybody, it being of no repute to act kindly and graciously and forbearingly only when receiving like treatment.

"They challenge all the world of industry to find a precept that could ever work better than 'Love thy neighbour as thyself' remembering always that God is Father of all.

"Therefore they desire to set out on this great adventure and as world citizens maintain friendly service, not only between themselves but towards all with whom they come in contact.

"To this end they are pursuing the following policy:

(1) To develop the strength of the Company.
(2) To benefit the members and employees of the Company.
(3) To produce goods beneficial to their customers at a fair price and of as high a quality as possible.

(4) To discharge their responsibility to the community, particularly in W—— and its neighbourhood.

(5) To conduct research and provide technical education in synthetic resins and their application in the paint, plastics and allied industries.

"The Common Ownership Constitution embodying these principles was unanimously adopted at the inaugural general meeting of the Company on the 28th April, in the year of the Festival of Britain 1951."

In the more than twenty years since this philosophy was introduced, accepted though at times questioned, the Company turnover has increased from £400,000 per annum to more than £6 million. As it has been put to me, while they have always to satisfy their shareholders there remains the very human desire to "share the cake", which means all the problems of industrial relations have constantly to be coped with. Nevertheless, such a philosophy can pay its way even in a highly competitive industry.

Our population can be divided into recognisable though heterogeneous groups, each of which seem to reflect a specific need or form of care. We may start with the adequate and inadequate, those able to care for themselves and those who need possibly several forms of specialised assistance. Then we have the age groups of infants (0–3), school children (3–13), adolescents (13–18), young adults (18–40), the middle-aged (40–65) and the elderly (65 +). Again we see the social classes and income groups. Through all these we can find the drones and the gluttons for work. Here there is the longest and shallowest gradient between the two extremes, which may be uneven, interrupted and reversible, a gradient governed by a host of factors, many of which I have touched upon in earlier chapters. In these groups and sub-groups there is a continuous flux, mostly progressive, as for instance with age and adequacy, but there may be from time to time regression, occasionally prolonged and illustrated by severe disablement, alcoholism or a long prison sentence.

The design and delivery of medical and social care for the population of this country continues to rest in the hands of different authorities both at central and local government level, resulting in gaps and duplications. The gaps are perhaps most obvious in the field of care and support of disabled people, in the rehabilitation of the mentally and physically sick, in the research and care of the socially ill population and in the vigilance of the health of those at work.

In this book we have been concerned with the last of these. Sometimes it is good, most times it is non-existent. The proportion of the population actually at work probably has not changed over the centuries, although one suspects that with the growing school, college and university population at one pole and the ageing people at the other, the proportion of the actual productive population on which the gross national product depends is becoming correspondingly less.

Very shortly the National Health Service is to be reorganised in an attempt to exclude some of the anomalies and deficiencies of health care. At the same time the responsibility of the Department of Employment towards the health of people at work has been very slightly broadened by the reorganisation of the pre-existing statutory Medical Inspectorate of Factories and Appointed Factory Doctor Service into the new Employment Medical Advisory Service.

The service came into operation on 1st February 1973 and will support the Factory Inspectorate; it will also answer specific inquiries concerning the physical working conditions of individual firms. From time to time the Employment Medical Advisory Service will request help from employers in carrying out investigations or research into problems of health of people at work.

The new service in no way obviates the present industrial medical services supported and maintained by public and private industry, but will complement them by the provision of professional advice and specialised facilities if requested. The embodying Act made this point quite clearly and stated that its policy was to support and encourage the existing industrial medical services.

Nevertheless, the new service will not be able to do more than meet minimal demands in view of the restricted number of medical and more serious, nursing personnel. It is envisaged that there will be about a hundred full-time doctor equivalents and 11 full-time nurse equivalents for the whole country. The emphasis placed on the nurse in industry by many industry-supported occupational health services indicates that it is in this field that the day-to-day occupational health monitoring takes place, by qualified nursing staff familiar with plant and personnel, backed by doctors with special training and understanding of the pattern of local industry. The new government service fails to provide a continuing human and environmental monitoring. There has been considerable disagreement between government advisers and experienced occupational health workers in this respect, based perhaps on the realisation by the former of the need to take into account the total organisation of health services before applying additional resources in one particular field.

It has become clear that for a number of reasons the degree or load of individual ill-health among the working population has

M

fallen, although the national sickness absence figures show not only a total rise but also an increase in the frequency of short absences. Interpreting from this changing pattern, we can understand the increased need for "minor medicine" which has progressively heaped upon the shoulders of general practitioners in demands for certification to support the claim for sickness absence pay. The failure of the doctors to marry these demands to a realistic understanding of the interplay between the environment and conditions of their patients at work, at home and at leisure, has led inevitably to irresponsible certification which has hampered the industrial growth of this country. Significantly, too, it has kept the standard of living for most people behind that of our competitors.

I do not advocate as a practical proposition that all general practitioners should become occupational health trained, and engage in the preventive aspects of this work. The distribution of industry, the intricate commuting patterns of workers and a host of other factors would make this unnecessary. Yet something could be done to reduce the reliance upon uninformed certification. Perhaps, taking the experience of both industrially developed communist countries and the still only partially developed countries attempting to build up their industries, the idea of primary health care at or near the place of work is worth attention. Last year (1972) a lively correspondence arose in the medical press following the publication of a critical report of British general practice by an American research worker. His main concern was with standards but he also examined the delivery of services to the various groups in the general community, one of these being working men in industry. His remark that ". . . the data available strongly suggest the need for an industrial medical service to give men easier access to medical care" should be carefully examined.

Men seek the advice of a general practitioner less often than women, important factors being the nature of men's work, the distance of work from the home, and the nature of and the patient's sensitivity to his disabilities, in particular the absence of gynaecological disorders. In addition, working women who have access to occupational health services have higher attendance rates than men and may take more readily the advice of the nursing or medical authorities to seek early treatment from their general practitioner. Only 10 per cent of our working population have access to occupational health services, but this could be a significant factor in areas where services do exist.

Convenience of attendance is important, and it is probably true that women tend to work nearer home than men. General practice reorganisation has not improved the ease of access for working men, who may lose up to a day's work, and pay, to attend the doctor for something they may regard as trivial. This has an analogy within the occupational health service – those clinics on site having higher attendance rates than those at some distance from the work-site.

The occupational health doctor has constantly to remind himself that he must not transgress the boundaries of the general practitioner's responsibility. He is nevertheless aware that quick and available advice for something quite unrelated to a man's work – for instance, a football injury over the weekend – may result in rapid reduction in symptoms and quicker healing, at the same time possibly eliminating the need to call on the general practitioner or the local hospital casualty department. This is in accord with his responsibility to make a diagnosis if possible and then refer the patient to his general practitioner. The constant presence of a medical unit at a man·s work, whether in a large company or through a group service, could do much to reduce the problem of unrecognised illness and improve early diagnosis, not only assisting the patient's comfort but also reducing the appalling level of sickness absence in Britain.

The one organisational argument which can be levelled against a work-based primary medical care service is that, in the event of major illness requiring long-term absence from work or even hospita-lisation, the doctor at work would not be in a position to undertake on-going care. While the reality of this is appreciated, it is not necessarily inhibitory to the idea of work-based medical care because, with modern means of communication, the local situation can be dealt with by referral to a local physician in the patient's home area by an emergency attendance or home visit. This is constantly happening in the work situation: the general practitioner is contacted for both occupationally induced and non-occupational illnesses.

With a general acceptance of the concept of the care of workers at work by community doctors the above suggestions could become reality, as they already have in areas where the general practitioners have a special interest in the occupational health care of workers in local industries. The awareness by general practitioners of their responsibility to workers at work, whether in shop, office, laboratory or production unit, must be stressed. The dissociated pattern of medical care in this country is at the root of a lot of needless delay in diagnosis, minor suffering and major sickness absence. I am not saying that primary medical care of workers should be taken away from the general practitioner: I am suggesting that consideration be given to putting the responsibility for the total health care of the full-time worker in the hands of work-based general practitioners with special interest in occupational health near his place of work.

There is no question that the traditional – in the sense of "currently accepted" – form of occupational health, particularly in the minds of those who make and interpret our laws, plays an important part in the daily lives of all of us by the standards set and with which firms and individuals are expected to comply. But the physical ill-effects of work play only a very small part in our overall morbidity (see Table 1).

TABLE 1

COMPARATIVE LOSS FROM SICKNESS, ACCIDENTS AND STRIKES DAYS (MILLIONS) LOST JUNE 1970–71

	Males	Females	Total
Certified sickness	244·64	69·49	314·13
Work accidents	16·63	2·45	19·08
Prescribed industrial disease	0·6	0·25	0·85
Strikes			13·551

The mental effects of human behaviour at work and elsewhere, whether they result in stupid accidents, poor industrial morale or overt psychiatric illness, exert an enormous influence.

These seemingly heretical views could be aligned with the stated philosophy behind the Employment Medical Advisory Service. Along with doctors undertaking primary medical care adjacent to work-sites, the service could provide specialist support and further investigation of work-induced injury or illness. This is unlikely to happen in the near future principally because of the professional isolation of doctors in the new service from those in active clinical practice in the National Health Service. However, the absorption of the Employment Medical Advisory Service within the National Health Service has not been ruled out by the present government, but it is recognised that its first job is to develop a worthwhile service to industry and achieve acceptance and co-operation from the other medical services: absorption within the National Health Service at this time would swamp its effectiveness as a new tool.

Health and happiness are not to be obtained at the hands of the doctors alone, a tradition that has ruled for less than a hundred years. Until the middle of the nineteenth century people took active steps to avoid doctors and hospitals which they considered to be pest-holes, with some justification – sentiments echoed by Molière, George Bernard Shaw and others.

The well-being of us all is subject to many influences, but the self-discipline we impose upon ourselves is paramount. Undisciplined lives lead, sooner or later, to ill-health and unhappiness. The moral issues in our lives has been exercising the attention of many people who are aware of the steady decline in personal and community responsibility which has been abrogated to government agencies. Prof. Tredgold of University College Hospital has recently emphasised the frustration and emotional conflicts which appear to be so much a part of our daily lives when he says that ". . . What we are seeing in industry is a reflection of what is going on in society. As individuals used to work in the past to resolve their emotional conflicts, so society today is using industry to solve its crises. Can doctors help? Presumably only by increasing the awareness of society as to what it is doing, as to what possible outlets it may choose, and their consequences." Across the Atlantic the picture is put differently but no less thoughtfully in the manner of Americans who are brought up to expect, in the immortal words of their constitution, that "life, liberty and the pursuit of happiness" are theirs by right of statute. Dr. John S. Millis, the President and Director of the United States National Fund for Medical Education, has recently asked "Can society promise health?" "The great health problems of the United States are not so much those of episodic illness as they are problems of personal behaviour. The greatest cause of both morbidity and mortality of Americans between the ages of one and thirty-seven is automobile accidents. It is reported that the elimination of obesity would increase our life expectancy by six years. We know that lung cancer and emphysema (ballooning of the lungs) are related to cigarette smoking. Alcoholism affects millions of people. Drug abuse is endemic. Millions of our citizens live emotionally un-disciplined lives with disastrous consequences to their health and life expectancy. Few of these problems are particularly affected by the availability of physicians, hospitals, clinics or nursing homes. No programme of national health insurance will protect people from the consequences of their behaviour. It will only be useful after the fact – to deal with illness much of which should never occur".

Bibliography

1. *Health in Industry: a Guide for Engineers, Executives and Doctors.* By R. C. Browne. London, 1961, p. 157.
2. *Industrial Health and Technology.* By Brian Harvey and Robert Murray. London, 1958, p. 337.
3. *De Re Metallica.* By Agricola (George Bauer). Translated by H. C. and L. H. Hoover. London, 1912.
4. *Safety and Health at Work.* Report of the Committee, 1970–72. Chairman, Lord Robens. H.M.S.O., 1972, p. 218.
5. *The Diseases of Occupations.* By Donald Hunter. 5th Edition. London, 1969, p. 1259.
6. *Human Documents of the Industrial Revolution in Britain.* By E. Royston Pike. London, 1966, p. 368.
7. *The National Atlas of Disease Mortality in the United Kingdom.* By G. Melvyn Howe. London, 1970, p. 197.
8. *Rehabilitation.* Report of the Sub-committee of the Standing Medical Advisory Committee. Chairman, Sir Ronald Tunbridge. H.M.S.O., 1972, p. 187.
9. *Social Psychology of Industry.* By J. A. C. Brown. London, 1954, p. 330.
10. *Prescribed Industrial Diseases.* Department of Health and Social Security, NI 2. January 1972.
11. *Occupational Health Practice.* Ed. R. S. F. Schilling. London, 1973, p. 466.

MINOR REFERENCES

1. *Ergonomics.* New South Wales Department of Public Health, Division of Occupational Health. Sydney, 1970, p. 17.
2. "Borderlines of Medicine and Ecology". By Sir Frank Fraser

Darling. *Proceedings of the Royal Society of Medicine*, 63. pp. 1164–67. 1970.

3. Letter to the *Daily Telegraph*. From John Rogers. 31st December 1970.

4. *When Violence becomes the Bedfellow of Boredom*. By John Bosworth. *Daily Telegraph*, 13th October 1969.

5. "The Challenge of the Painful Back". By A. Maxwell Robertson. *Transactions of Society of Occupational Medicine*, 20. 1970, pp. 42–9.

6. "Six Cases of Acrylamide Poisoning". By T. O. Garland and M. W. H. Patterson. *British Medical Journal*, 4. 1967, pp. 134–8.

7. "Alcoholism in Scotland." By Martin Whittet. *Transactions of the Society of Occupational Medicine*, 20. 1970, pp. 119–26.

8. *Aldrin, Dieldrin, Endrin and Telodrin*. By K. W. Jager. Amsterdam, 1970, p. 234.

9. "Determination of Zinc in Biological Fluids." By A. S. Prasad, D. Oberleas and J. A. Halstead in *Zinc Metabolism*. Springfield, Illinois, 1966.

10. "Aspects of the Genetical Theory of the Inborn Errors of Metabolism." By H. Harris. *Triangle*, 10. 1971, pp. 41–6.

11. "Rehabilitation of the Coronary Patient." By T. Semple. *Transactions of the Society of Occupational Medicine*, 18. 1968, pp. 135–41.

12. *Trader Horn*. By Alfred Aloysius Horn. London, 1932, p. 310.

13. *Medicine in Modern Society*. By T. McKeown. London, 1965, p. 234.

14. *The Prevention of Malaria in the Federated Malay States*. By Malcolm Watson. Liverpool, 1911, p. 139.

15. *Kuwait: Urban and Medical Ecology*. By G. E. Ffrench and A. G. Hill. Berlin, 1971, p. 122.

16. "Quality in General Practice." By Frank Honigsbaum. *Journal of the Royal College of General Practitioners*, 22. 1972, pp. 429–51.

17. "Insecurity in Industry." By R. F. Tredgold. *Proceedings of the Royal Society of Medicine*, 65. 1972, pp. 1087–9.

18. "Can Security Promise Health." By John S. Millis. *Linacre Quarterly*, 39. 1972, p. 80–3.

Index

Spine 49 et seq.
Status 32
Stoke-Manderville Hospital 128
Strikes 160
Student Health 33, 146
Styrene 146
Submarines 53
Sulpha drugs 72
Sussex 3
Sweden 13, 19, 145
Syphilis 154
Syrian legionaries 15

Talc 85
Taylor, E. J. 24
Taylor, Peter 48
Tea 109
Ten Hours Bill 24
Teratogenic effects 107
Textiles 5
Thermopolyspora polyspora 147
Thirty Years War 13
Threshold Limit Value 73
Tin 85
Trade Unions 10, 23, 39, 40
Training 6, 34, 56
Transport and General Workers Union 135
Transportation 38
Treaty of Rome 7
Tredgold, Professor 171
Trinidad 158
Trollope, Anthony 155
Trotter, Thomas 75

T- total 77
Tuberculosis 69, 74
Tunbridge Report 124, 126

Underdeveloped countries 22
United States 22, 77, 81, 82, 109
Unity of command 23, 24, 27
University 3, 33, 38
University College Hospital 171

Vanadium 85, 106, 107, 146
Vaughan, David 143
Vicea fava 149
Viruses 122, 158
Vitamins 107, 108

Wadi Batin 158, 160
War 5, 9, 10, 13, 52, 53, 157
Watson, Sir Malcolm 157, 158
Weald 3
Welfare 7, 15, 22
West Country 3
West Midlands (Birmingham) Industrial Health Service 10
Whittet, Dr. Martin 82
Widowed 81
Women 5, 21, 35, 36, 41, 57
Woodworkers 95

X-ray 73, 93, 143, 147

Yellow Fever 158
Yorkshire 21, 25, 61

Zinc 98, 99, 106, 109